Laboratory

Indices of

Nutritional

Status in

Pregnancy

Committee on Nutrition of the Mother and
  Preschool Child
Food and Nutrition Board
National Research Council

NATIONAL ACADEMY OF SCIENCES
Washington, D.C.   1978

NOTICE: The project that is the subject of this report was approved by the Governing Board of the National Research Council, whose members are drawn from the Councils of the National Academy of Sciences, the National Academy of Engineering, and the Institute of Medicine. The members of the Committee responsible for the report were chosen for their special competences and with regard for appropriate balance.

This report has been reviewed by a group other than the authors according to procedures approved by a Report Review Committee consisting of members of the National Academy of Sciences, the National Academy of Engineering, and the Institute of Medicine.

The study summarized in this report was supported by Grant MC-R-110354-02-0 from the Bureau of Community Health Services, PHS-DHEW.

Available from:
Printing and Publishing Office
National Academy of Sciences
2101 Constitution Avenue, N.W.
Washington, D.C. 20418

Printed in the United States of America

COMMITTEE ON NUTRITION OF THE MOTHER AND PRESCHOOL CHILD

ROY M. PITKIN, *Chairman*
VIRGINIA A. BEAL
FRANK FALKNER
PERRY A. HENDERSON
JANET C. KING
ALVIN M. MAUER
W. ANN REYNOLDS
ROBERT E. SHANK
WILLIAM N. SPELLACY
MERVYN W. SUSSER

NAS-NRC Staff Officer: MYRTLE L. BROWN

iii

Preface

Pregnancy is characterized by extensive maternal physiologic adjustments involving a variety of metabolic processes. These characteristic changes are often reflected in altered results of laboratory tests such that values in healthy pregnant women may fall outside a "normal range" derived from studies of nonpregnant individuals. Failure to appreciate the effects of normal gestation can thus result in errors in diagnosis.

The primary purpose of this publication is to review the current state of knowledge regarding laboratory indices reflecting nutritional and metabolic status during normal pregnancy and thus provide normative data with respect to such indices in the healthy gravida. A secondary aim is to identify gaps and deficiencies in understanding of this fundamental aspect of human biology.

Because maternal physiologic adjustments represent a dynamic process, special care has been taken, insofar as possible with existing data, to tabulate values with respect to the duration of gestation. Consideration has been limited to the antepartum period (i.e., excluding parturition and the puerperium), and no effort has been made to include abnormalities or disease states.

The book was prepared under the auspices and supervision of the Committee on Nutrition of the Mother and Preschool Child, a committee of the Food and Nutrition Board, National Research Council. Each of its seven chapters was written by an individual or individuals with special expertise in the particular field, assisted in many cases by review and consultation with a working group of other experts.

Support for the Committee's activities, including this publication, has been provided by the Bureau of Community Health Services, U.S. Department of Health, Education, and Welfare. Additional financial assistance was provided by Ross Laboratories, Columbus, Ohio.

Contents

vii

1

Physiologic Adjustments in General

ROY M. PITKIN *and* WILLIAM N. SPELLACY

BODY WEIGHT AND COMPOSITION

The magnitude and patterns of weight gain during pregnancy have been the subject of much study over many years. Nevertheless, definition of normative data is beset with great difficulty. After reviewing 35 published reports dealing with weight gain over at least the last two-thirds of gestation, Hytten and Leitch (1971) concluded that few if any met acceptable criteria for establishment of normality. Among the deficiencies of these reports were: (1) manipulation of weight, usually by advice to restrict the diet; (2) failure to differentiate between normal and abnormal pregnancies; (3) questionable reliability of the prepregnant weight; and (4) inability to assess potential modifying influences such as age, parity, and antecedent body weight. Thus, it is not possible to determine normal values with any degree of confidence in their precision. At best, only estimates of the average pattern can be made. Moreover, in any population there will be a considerable distribution about this average.

Total weight gain during pregnancy probably averages between 10 and 12 kg (Pitkin *et al.*, 1972). Customarily, there is minimal change during the early weeks following conception. Near the end of the first trimester, weight begins to accrue, and gain continues until parturition. Individual subjects exhibit considerable variability, but in general the

1

rate of gain during the second and third trimesters is essentially linear and averages 350 to 400 g/wk. While great emphasis has been placed on *total* weight gain, it seems self-evident that the *pattern* by which weight accumulates is the more important datum.

The pattern and components of gestational weight gain, using data from several sources, are illustrated in Figure 1-1. If total gain is assumed to be 11 kg at term, the maternal compartment represents 6 kg and the fetal compartment 5 kg. While the overall rate of gain is similar over the last two trimesters, accumulation in maternal and fetal compartments varies with stage of pregnancy. During the second trimester, most of the gain reflects increase of maternal components with blood volume expansion, growth of uterus and breasts, and storage of fat. By contrast, during the third trimester most of the growth involves the fetus, placenta, and amniotic fluid, while maternal tissues and fluids (except for extracellular fluid) increase to only a small degree.

Determinations of body composition in pregnancy necessarily reflect the combination of the maternal organism and the products of conception. Moreover, the opportunity for direct analysis in the human

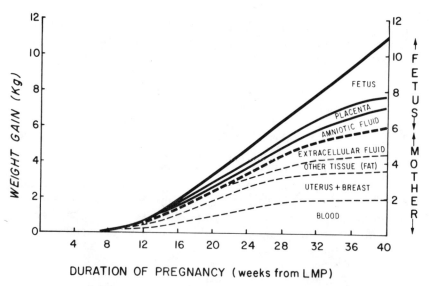

DURATION OF PREGNANCY (weeks from LMP)

FIGURE 1-1 Pattern and components of cumulative gain in weight during pregnancy assuming total gain of 11 kg. Reproduced with permission from Pitkin (1976).

virtually never exists, and it is necessary to rely on indirect (e.g., isotope dilution) indices. Total body water increases progressively; several deuterium oxide studies summarized by Hytten and Leitch (1971) indicate an increment of about 7 l by term. Most of this accumulation, 5 or 6 l, reflects extracellular water. However, pregnant women with edema (particularly generalized) may have substantially greater amounts. Fat increase during pregnancy, evidenced by under-water weighing and measurement of skinfold thickness, averages ap-proximately 2 kg but is highly variable. The total amount of protein added during pregnancy, calculated from nitrogen measurements of fetus, placenta, and expanded maternal components, amounts to slightly less than 1 kg. Whether protein is stored in additional sites, such as liver and muscle, is a matter of considerable controversy (King, 1975). Sodium and other minerals accumulate in amounts ap-propriate to the added tissues and fluids of mother and fetus, but their contribution to total weight is minimal.

ENDOCRINE ACTIVITY

Pregnancy is associated with elaboration of peptide and steroid hor-mones having effects extending beyond the reproductive system. Many of the physiologic adjustments discussed throughout this publication result directly or indirectly from these pregnancy hormones, the serum levels of which are illustrated in Figures 1-2 through 1-5. Because of methodological variation, the illustrations are intended to depict gen-eral trends rather than absolute values.

Human chorionic gonadotropin (HCG) (Figure 1-2) may be detected in the serum and urine within a few days after implantation. Because of its close chemical, immunological, and biological relationship to pitui-tary luteinizing hormone, most assay systems do not differentiate these two agents. Recent developments of radioimmunoassays utilizing only the beta subunit of the HCG molecule, however, permit clear distinc-tion. Serum levels increase rapidly during early pregnancy to peak values at approximately 60 days after conception. Thereafter, they decline as quickly as they rose until a relatively low level is reached, which is then maintained until term. The principal reproductive effect of HCG is maintenance of the corpus luteum in early pregnancy, providing hormonal support of the developing conceptus until placental steroid production becomes sufficient. HCG has few known effects on nonreproductive tissues.

Human placental lactogen (HPL) (Figure 1-3) is synthesized by the

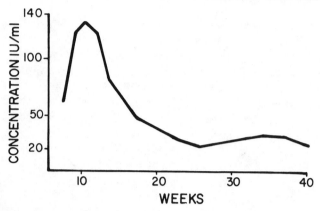

FIGURE 1-2 Pattern of human chorionic gonadotropin (HCG) levels in serum during pregnancy. Based on data of Teoh (1967).

syncytiotrophoblast in progressively increased amounts during pregnancy. Its precise role in reproduction is poorly understood, but, based on its marked immunologic and biologic similarity with growth hormone, it may represent some type of growth factor for the fetus and/or placenta. In any event, serum levels seem to correlate with placental

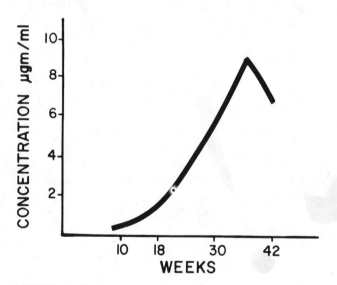

FIGURE 1-3 Pattern of human placental lactogen (HPL) during pregnancy. Based on data of Spellacy (1972).

mass and to be raised or lowered with certain types of pregnancy complications. HPL exerts effects on carbohydrate and lipid metabolism and seems to be a major factor in the pregnancy adjustments reviewed in detail in Chapter 4.

All three classical estrogens (estrone, estradiol, and estriol) increase during the pregnancy (Figure 1-4). The initial source of estrogens is the corpus luteum, maintained for the early weeks after conception by HCG. Estrogen biosynthesis during the last two-thirds of gestation is a complicated process involving coordinated activities by mother, fetus, and placenta. In addition to its considerable effects on the uterus and other reproductive organs, estrogen exerts more generalized influences. It produces a rise in concentration of certain binding proteins, particularly those globulins that bind hormones, with the result that total hormone levels are elevated, while amounts of unbound (and biologically active) hormone remain unchanged. Estrogen also appears to be involved to some extent in adjustments in carbohydrate and lipid metabolism during pregnancy.

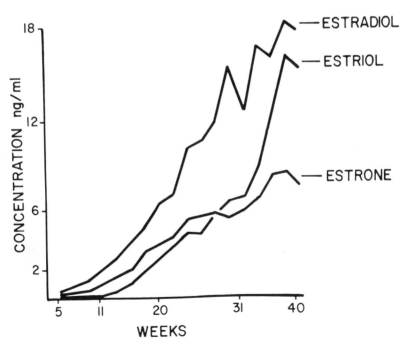

FIGURE 1-4   Pattern of estrone, estradiol, and estriol in serum during pregnancy. Based on data of deHertogh *et al.* (1975).

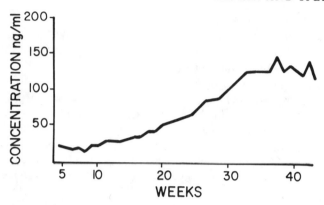

FIGURE 1-5   Pattern of progesterone in plasma during pregnancy.
Based on data of Johansson (1969).

Progesterone levels rise progressively during pregnancy (Figure 1-5).
The initial source is the corpus luteum, but later placental sources
come to predominate. Progestational effects include relaxation of
smooth muscle, not only of the genital tract but of other organs as well.
Thus, the tendency to atony of the gastrointestinal and urinary tracts
appears to be a reflection of progesterone influence.

ORGAN SYSTEMS

A number of changes in the cardiovascular system accompany pregnancy. Pulse rate increases by an average of 15 to 20 beats/min to a
maximum in the early third trimester and falls slightly thereafter.
Arterial blood pressure, particularly the diastolic component, falls
through the first and second trimesters and then rises during the last
trimester to reach the nonpregnant levels by term. The effect of
pregnancy on cardiac output is a matter of some controversy, but it
seems likely that the fall in late pregnancy described in earlier studies
reflected inferior vena cava obstruction and that the increased level of
pregnancy persists from at least midgestation until term. The increased
cardiac output amounts to about a third of nonpregnant norms (4.5 to
6.0 l/min) while that of pulse rate is but a fifth (70 to 85 beats/min); thus,
a small rise in stroke volume must also occur. Venous pressure
centrally and in the upper extremity is unaffected by pregnancy, while
that of the lower extremity rises progressively with advancing
gestation.

In respiratory function, the vital capacity is unchanged but its components are rearranged. Tidal volume increases, mainly at the expense of expiratory reserve volume, and this change, coupled with a diminished residual volume, leads to the gravida's lung being, in effect, more collapsed at the end of expiration. Gas mixing in the lung is thus more efficient. Alveolar pCO_2 falls during the luteal phase of the cycle, and this progesterone effect continues into and through pregnancy.

Renal changes of two types, anatomic and functional, accompany pregnancy. The principal anatomic effect is dilation of the renal pelvis and ureter, typically with a right-sided preponderance. At first the mechanism was assumed to be mechanical, but this was replaced by a hormonal (progesterone) theory; the bulk of recent evidence seems to favor a primary mechanical cause with additive endocrine effects. Renal plasma flow seems to be increased by some 200 to 250 ml/min from early pregnancy onwards. Similarly, glomerular filtration rate is elevated by as much as 50 percent throughout at least the last two-thirds of gestation. Such changes have profound implications with respect to urinary clearance, as discussed in detail in other sections. The activity of the renin-angiotensin system is greatly enhanced during pregnancy. The concentrations of renin and renin substrate are both increased severalfold. The increased angiotensin levels, which would be the anticipated result, do not, however, result in elevation of arterial blood pressure because of the high degree of angiotensin resistance exhibited by the pregnant woman. Thus, the major physiologic consequence of increased angiotensin activity production appears to be stimulation of aldosterone secretion, which enhances tubular reabsorption of sodium and other substances from the glomerular filtrate.

The major effect of pregnancy on the alimentary tract is a generalized reduction in tone and motility of the stomach and small and large intestines, presumably a reflection of the smooth-muscle relaxing property of progesterone. As a result, gastric emptying and intestinal transit times are prolonged. Gastric acid secretion is fairly regularly reduced and the incidence of achlorhydria correspondingly increased. Liver function is generally unaffected by pregnancy, although certain "liver function tests" (e.g., a fall in serum albumin or a rise in alkaline phosphatase due to increased heat-stable enzyme from the placenta) exhibit characteristic alterations.

REFERENCES

deHertogh, R., K. Thomas, Y. Bietlot, I. Vanderheyden, and J. Ferin. 1975. Plasma levels of unconjugated estrone, estradiol, and estriol and of HCS throughout pregnancy in normal women. J. Clin. Endocrinol. Metab. 40:93–101.

Hytten, F. E., and I. Leitch. 1971. The Physiology of Human Pregnancy, 2d ed. Blackwell Scientific Publications, Oxford. 599 pp.

Johansson, E. D. B. 1969. Plasma levels of progesterone in pregnancy measured by a rapid competitive protein binding technique. Acta Endocrinol. 61:607–617.

King, J. C. 1975. Protein metabolism in pregnancy. Clin. Perinatol. 2:243–254.

Pitkin, R. M. 1976. Nutritional support in obstetrics and gynecology. Clin. Obstet. Gynecol. 19:489–513.

Pitkin, R. M., H. A. Kaminetzky, M. Newton, and J. A. Pritchard. 1972. Maternal nutrition: a selective review of clinical topics. Obstet. Gynecol. 40:773–785.

Spellacy, W. N. 1972. Immunoassay of human placental lactogen: physiological studies in normal and abnormal pregnancy, pp. 223–239. In G. E. W. Wolstenholme and J. Knight, ed., Ciba Foundation Symposium on Lactogenic Hormones. London, 1971.

Teoh, E. S. 1967. Chorionic gonadotrophin in the serum and urine of Asian women in normal pregnancy. J. Obstet. Gynaecol. Br. Commonw. 74:74–79.

2

Hematologic Indices

ROY M. PITKIN

ROY M. PITKIN

HEMOGLOBIN-ERYTHROCYTE INDICES

As summarized in the preceding chapter, an increasing maternal blood volume represents one of the fundamental physiologic adjustments of pregnancy. The pattern of change differs substantially for plasma and erythrocytes, and this difference accounts for alterations in various hemoglobin-erythrocyte indices during the course of gestation. The increase in plasma volume follows a gently sigmoid pattern with the increase beginning in the first trimester, continuing through the second and early third trimesters, and then leveling off during the last 6–8 wk of pregnancy. At maximum, the augmented plasma volume amounts to an average of 1,200 ml, or approximately 50 percent of the nonpregnant mean (Hytten and Paintin, 1963). Total erythrocyte volume, by contrast, exhibits a more nearly linear pattern of increase, which at term attains a value some 20 to 30 percent above that of the nonpregnant (Hytten and Leitch, 1971).

As a consequence of these differential rates of increase for plasma and erythrocytes, the hemoglobin concentration, hematocrit, and erythrocyte count decline during pregnancy, reaching a nadir at 32–34 wk and rising slightly thereafter. While the general pattern of these changes is not particularly influenced by maternal iron status, the absolute levels depend directly on this variable.

9

Table 2-1 contains values from a number of different studies of hemoglobin concentration, hematocrit or packed cell volume, erythrocyte count, mean corpuscular volume (MCV), mean corpuscular hemoglobin (MCH), and mean corpuscular hemoglobin concentration (MCHC). All studies were longitudinal in nature. Table 2-1 is arranged by gestational duration and by presence or absence of iron supplementation.

It can be seen that the hemoglobin concentration, hematocrit, and erythrocyte count decline progressively, particularly in unsupplemented subjects in which mean values at mid-third trimester are usually in the range of 10.5 to 11.0 g/dl for hemoglobin, 32 to 34 percent for hematocrit, and 3.7 to 4.1 million/mm^3 for erythrocyte count. Iron supplementation "blunts" this response so that mean values during the mid-third trimester are usually about 12 g/dl for hemoglobin, 36 percent for hematocrit, and 4 million/mm^3 for erythrocyte count. Further evidence of the effect of iron on hemoglobin indices may be found in the review by Pritchard (1970), in which the mean hemoglobin concentration at or near term in five reported studies was 12.3 g/dl with iron supplements and 11.1 g/dl without.

As indicated additionally in Table 2-1, neither the volume nor the hemoglobin content of individual erythrocytes change remarkably during gestation, nor does iron supplementation have an appreciable influence. However, the concentration of hemoglobin within individual erythrocytes is increased slightly in women taking iron supplements.

A diurnal variation in hematocrit, with higher values in the morning than in the afternoon, has been described during the third trimester of pregnancy (Agboola, 1974). The diurnal change was slight, though statistically significant, averaging 0.7 vol%.

The reticulocyte count apparently increases during pregnancy, presumably reflecting increased erythropoietic activity. In a study of healthy, nonanemic, iron-sufficient Anglo-Saxon women in the third trimester, the mean value was 1.2 percent (range, 0.2–1.8 percent), compared with a 6 wk postpartum mean of 0.8 percent (Traill, 1975). Higher reticulocyte counts were found in women of Greek and Italian descent, even though hemolytic anemia had been ruled out in all subjects.

Erythrocyte fragility, customarily expressed as the strength of saline solution at which hemolysis of 50 percent of erythrocytes occurs, increases during pregnancy to a maximum at 32 wk and declines slightly thereafter. For example, in a longitudinal study of 22 patients examined at 4-wk intervals, Robertson (1968) found values of 0.432

percent at 8 wk, 0.460 percent at 32 wk, and 0.451 percent at term. The increase in erythrocyte fragility presumably reflects the fall in serum colloid osmotic pressure due to fall in serum proteins and is of no pathological significance.

LEUKOCYTE INDICES

The total leukocyte count increases during pregnancy. Values from two reports (both cross-sectional investigations) are listed in Table 2-2. Though somewhat different values were found in these studies, there is agreement that the mean count apparently rises shortly after conception to a level near the traditional upper limit of normal for the nonpregnant ($10,000/mm^3$) and changes little throughout the remainder of pregnancy.

The cell type mainly responsible for the leukocytosis of pregnancy is the neutrophil, with the result that the mean proportion of the total leukocyte count represented by phagocytic cells rises from 66 percent in nonpregnant to 76 percent in pregnant subjects (Mitchell *et al.*, 1966). Eosinophils, basophils, and monocytes change little if any during gestation, while the lymphocyte count declines by 10–15 percent from the first to the third trimester (Efrati *et al.*, 1964).

Published data regarding counts of the types of leukocytes in pregnancy all relate to relative proportions rather than absolute numbers. In view of the increase in both total leukocyte count and relative proportion of neutrophils, the absolute neutrophil count would be expected to increase substantially. Similarly, eosinophils, basophils, and monocytes should not change relatively, but should increase absolutely. In the case of lymphocytes, a decline in percentage is balanced against a similar increase in total count; thus, the absolute number of lymphocytes per unit volume probably does not change appreciably during gestation.

The morphology of polymorphonuclear leukocytes, in particular the number of nuclear lobes per cell, is important because of the well-known tendency to neutrophil hypersegmentation with folate deficiency. Kitay *et al.* (1969) computed the average number of lobes in 100 consecutively observed leukocytes in peripheral blood smears; in 188 normal pregnant and puerperal subjects, the mean ($\pm SD$) value was 2.90 (± 0.36). This was statistically significantly less than that of 59 nonpregnant gynecologic patients (3.07 $\pm$ 0.32), indicating that pregnancy per se does not cause hypersegmentation. Neither parity nor duration of pregnancy exerted any influence on the lobe average.

TABLE 2-1 Hemoglobin-Erythrocyte Indices

References	Unsupplemented or Placebo									Iron Supplements (78–115 mg/d)								
	12 wk	16 wk	20 wk	24 wk	28 wk	32 wk	36 wk	40 wk	PP	12 wk	16 wk	20 wk	24 wk	28 wk	32 wk	36 wk	40 wk	PP
Hemoglobin (g/dl)																		
DeLeeuw et al. (1966)	12.5	12.4	11.7	11.4	11.0	10.6	10.7	10.9	11.9	11.4	11.4	11.8	11.8	11.8	11.8	12.0	12.4	13.0
Chanarin et al. (1965)		12.9	12.2		11.8		11.8	12.0	12.1		12.8	12.0			12.1	12.4	13.0	13.1
Chanarin et al. (1968)											12.2				12.0	12.5		
Paintin et al. (1966)			11.7 (±0.7)		10.4 (±0.9)		10.7 (±1.0)		11.9 (±1.0)			11.6 (±0.8)		11.3 (±0.9)		12.0 (±1.0)		12.6 (±0.9)
Lind (1975)	12.2 (±0.8)				11.2 (±0.7)	11.1 (±0.8)	11.0 (±0.8)	11.1 (±0.9)		12.4 (±1.0)				11.4 (±1.0)	11.6 (±1.1)	11.7 (±1.3)	12.2 (±1.3)	
Svanberg et al. (1975)	12.5 (±0.13)	12.2 (±0.11)	11.6 (±0.12)	11.5 (±0.14)	11.3 (±0.14)	11.3 (±0.16)	11.4 (±0.17)		12.9 (±0.15)	12.5 (±0.18)	12.0 (±0.14)	11.6 (±0.14)	11.6 (±0.17)	11.6 (±0.13)	12.0 (±0.17)	12.4 (±0.18)		13.4 (±0.18)
Hematocrit (vol %)																		
DeLeeuw et al. (1966)	38.3	39.5	36.4	35.6	34.6	34.1	34.3	34.9	39.1	35.7	36.3	37.1	37.1	36.8	37.0	37.5	38.7	39.8
Chanarin et al. (1965)		39.1	37.3		36.7	36.7	36.7	36.9	37.7		38.9	36.7			36.9	37.9	39.1	40.0
Chanarin et al. (1965)											37			36	36	38		
Lind (1975)	35.3 (±2.4)				32.7 (±2.3)	32.6 (±2.5)	32.6 (±2.3)	32.8 (±2.1)		36.0 (±2.5)				33.2 (±2.6)	34.0 (±3.0)	34.2 (±3.4)	36.0 (±3.4)	

12

Svanberg *et al.* (1975)	38.0 (±0.4)	37.0 (±0.4)	35.4 (±0.4)	35.3 (±0.4)	34.2 (±0.4)	34.2 (±0.5)	34.7 (±0.5)	39.9 (±0.4)	38.0 (±0.5)	36.4 (±0.4)	35.4 (±0.4)	35.4 (±0.5)	34.9 (±0.4)	36.6 (±0.5)	36.9 (±0.7)	40.5 (±0.5)
Erythrocytes (10⁶/mm³)																
DeLeeuw *et al.* (1966)	4.4	4.4	4.1	4.1	4.1	4.1	4.1	4.6	4.0	4.0	4.1	4.1	4.1	4.1	4.3	4.4
Lind (1975)	4.2 (±0.3)				3.7 (±0.3)	3.7 (±0.3)	3.8 (±0.3)	3.9 (±0.3)					3.8 (±0.3)	3.9 (±0.3)	3.9 (±0.3)	4.0 (±0.3)
MCV (u³)																
DeLeeuw *et al.* (1966)	86	90	90	90	89	89	90	91	90	91	91	91	91	90	91	92
Lind (1975)	84.6 (±4.2)				88.0 (±4.8)	87.0 (±4.9)	85.8 (±5.3)	85.2 (±6.0)	83.6 (±4.9)				87.6 (±6.9)	87.3 (±6.8)	87.3 (±6.7)	89.1 (±7.0)
MCH (pg)																
Lind (1975)	29.3 (±1.6)				30.3 (±1.6)	29.9 (±1.7)	29.1 (±2.1)	28.8 (±2.3)	28.9 (±2.1)				30.2 (±2.6)	30.0 (±2.6)	29.9 (±2.8)	30.4 (±2.8)
MCHC (%)																
DeLeeuw *et al.* (1966)	38	39	36	35	34	34	34	35	36	36	37	37	37	38	39	40
Paintin *et al.* (1966)			32.4 (±0.8)	32.4 (±1.0)	32.4 (±1.0)		31.6 (±1.4)	31.0 (±1.3)			32.3 (±0.9)		32.5 (±1.2)		32.2 (±1.3)	31.6 (±1.1)
Svanberg *et al.* (1975)	32.9 (±0.18)	33.0 (±0.19)	32.9 (±0.24)	32.6 (±0.18)	32.9 (±0.16)	32.7 (±0.18)	32.8 (±0.19)	32.3 (±0.24)	32.9 (±0.25)	33.0 (±0.19)	33.1 (±0.21)	33.0 (±0.29)	33.3 (±0.24)	32.8 (±0.19)	33.5 (±0.27)	33.1 (±0.19)

ᵃSix to thirteen weeks postpartum.

NOTE: All values refer to mean ± SEM except those of Lind, which are mean ± SD.

TABLE 2-2   Total Leukocyte Count $(10^3/mm^3)^a$

References	Nonpregnant Controls	Trimester		
		1	2	3
Efrati et al. (1964)		8.7	8.73	8.5
		(6.3–15)	(6.58–21.25)	(4–18)
Mitchell et al. (1966)	7.21	9.41	10.72	10.35
	(4.75–9.6)	(3.15–15.3)	(6.3–16.1)	(5–16.6)

^{a}Values are means with range in parentheses.

PLATELET AND COAGULATION INDICES

The effect of pregnancy on the platelet count is unclear. Sejeny et al. (1975) noted that, of 11 papers published from 1908 to 1968, 3 reported an increase, 3 a decrease, and 5 no significant change. This uncertainty is illustrated in the 4 reports listed in Table 2-3. It may be significant that the more recent studies, as well as the only longitudinal study, indicate a tendency (of varying proportions) for the platelet count to decline during gestation. Assuming that a decline does occur, its extent is no more (and perhaps less) than the increase in total blood volume. Thus the total platelet mass would remain constant or perhaps increase, a consideration of some physiologic significance, as the regulation of platelet production is thought to be indicated through total platelet mass rather than platelet count.

Fibrinogen has been studied extensively during pregnancy, and virtually all reports are in agreement that levels are generally increased over nonpregnant values, as indicated in Table 2-4. Discrepancies in absolute values among various reports probably reflect methodological differences. The exact point at which fibrinogen begins to rise is not entirely clear, but it increases progressively until term, at which the level is 100 mg/dl or more above nonpregnant norms, representing an increase of approximately 50 percent.

With respect to other coagulation factors, levels of factors VII and X increase by as much as fourfold and those of factors VIII and IX by 25 to 40 percent during gestation (Todd et al., 1965). By contrast, the concentrations of prothrombin and factors V, XI, and XII are unaffected (Todd et al., 1965).

Bleeding, clotting, and prothrombin times are unaffected by pregnancy (Margulis et al., 1954; Todd et al., 1965).

TABLE 2-3 Platelet Count ($10^3/mm^3$)

References	No. of Subjects	Type of Study	Nonpregnant Mean	Trimester		
				1	2	3
Mor et al. (1960)	200	Cross-sectional	187	210 (126–450)[a]	276 (126–639)[a]	316 (103–672)[a]
Sejeny et al. (1975)	405	Cross-sectional		210.4 ± 52.3[b]	203.3 ± 45.8[b]	183.9 ± 50.3[b]
Shaper et al. (1968)	20	Cross-sectional	236 ± 55[b,c]			172 ± 36[b]
Bonnar et al. (1969)	10	Longitudinal	250[c]	220	200	230

[a]Values in parentheses refer to observed range.
[b]Mean ± SD.
[c]Six week postpartum value.

15

TABLE 2-4   Plasma Fibrinogen Levels (mg/dl)

References	No. of Subjects	Type of Study	Nonpregnant Levels	Trimester		
				1	2	3
Bonnar et al. (1969)	10	Longitudinal	285^a	340	380	450
Todd et al. (1965)		Combined	322 ± 32^b	315	357	390
Shaper et al. (1968)	20	Cross-sectional	$350^a \pm 45^b$		432 $\pm 57^b$	

[a]Six week postpartum value.
[b]Mean ± SD.

REFERENCES

Agboola, A. 1974. Diurinal variation in hematocrit value in pregnancy. J. Obstet. Gynaecol. Br. Commonw. 81:901–902.
Bonnar, J., G. P. McNicol, and A. S. Douglas. 1969. Fibrinolytic enzyme system and pregnancy. Br. Med. J. 3:387–389.
Chanarin, I., D. Rothman, and V. Berry. 1965. Iron deficiency and its relation to folic-acid status in pregnancy: results of a clinical trial. Br. Med. J. 1:480–485.
Chanarin, I., D. Rothman, A. Ward, and J. Perry. 1968. Folate status and requirement in pregnancy. Br. Med. J. 2:390–397.
DeLeeuw, N. K. M., L. Lowenstein, and Y. Hsieh. 1966. Iron deficiency and hydremia in normal pregnancy. Medicine 45:291–315.
Efrati, P., B. Presentey, M. Margalith, and L. Rozenszajn. 1964. Leukocytes of normal pregnant women. Obstet. Gynecol. 23:429–432.
Hytten, F. E., and D. B. Paintin. 1963. Increase in plasma volume during normal pregnancy. J. Obstet. Gynaecol. Br. Commonw. 70:402–407.
Hytten, F. E., and I. Leitch. 1971. The Physiology of Human Pregnancy, 2d ed. Blackwell Scientific Publications, Oxford.
Kitay, D. J., W. J. Hogan, B. Eberle, and T. Mynt. 1969. Neutrophil hypersegmentation and folic acid deficiency in pregnancy. Am. J. Obstet. Gynecol. 104:1163–1173.
Lind T. 1975. Personal communication.
Margulis, R. R., J. H. Luzadre, and C. P. Hodgkinson. 1954. Fibrinolysis in labor and delivery. Obstet. Gynecol. 3:487–490.
Mitchell, A. W., Jr., R. J. McRipley, R. J. Selvaraz, and A. J. Sbarra. 1966. The role of the phagocyte in host-parasite interactions. IV. The phagocytic activity of leukocytes in pregnancy and its relationship to urinary tract infection. Am. J. Obstet. Gynecol. 96:687–695.
Mor, A., W. Yang, A. Schwartz, and W. C. Jones. 1960. Platelet counts in pregnancy and labor. Obstet. Gynecol. 16:338–343.
Paintin, D. B., A. M. Thomson, and F. E. Hytten. 1966. Iron and the haemoglobin level in pregnancy. J. Obstet. Gynaecol. Br. Commonw. 73:181–190.
Pritchard, J. A. 1970. Anemias complicating pregnancy and the puerperium, pp. 74–109. In Maternal Nutrition and the Course of Pregnancy. National Academy of Sciences, Washington, D.C.

Robertson, E. G. 1968. Increased erythrocyte fragility in association with osmotic changes in pregnancy serum. J. Reprod. Fertil. 16:323–324.

Sejeny, S. A., R. D. Eastham, and S. A. Baker. 1975. Platelet counts during normal pregnancy. J. Clin. Pathol. 28:812–813.

Shaper, A. G., J. Kear, D. M. Macintosh, J. Kyobe, and D. Njama. 1968. The platelet count, platelet adhesiveness and aggregation and the mechanism of fibrinolytic inhibition in pregnancy and the puerperium. J. Obstet. Gynaecol. Br. Commonw. 75:433–441.

Svanberg, B., B. Arvidson, A. Norrby, G. Rybo, and L. Solvell. 1975. Absorption of supplemental iron during pregnancy—a longitudinal study with repeated bone marrow and absorption measurements. Acta Obstet. Gynecol. Scand. Suppl. 48:87–108.

Todd, M. E., J. H. Thompson, Jr., E. J. W. Bowie, and C. A. Owen. 1965. Changes in blood coagulation during pregnancy. Mayo Clin. Proc. 40:370–383.

Traill, L. M. 1975. Reticulocytes in healthy pregnancy. Med. J. Aust. 2:205–206.

3

Electrolytes in
Normal Pregnancy

W. ANN REYNOLDS

Movement of electrolytes to and from plasma is governed by cell membranes throughout the body as well as by the kidneys. Intracellular fluid is characterized by high potassium and phosphate contents, while extracellular fluid normally contains high levels of sodium and chloride. Because of its quantity, its alterations with dietary intake, and its role in disease states, sodium is undoubtedly the most important cation, with potassium ranking second. It should be noted that inside the cell potassium is the principal cation, while sodium presides in interstitial fluid and serum. Similarly, chloride is the dominant anion; bicarbonate and phosphate are also important because of their buffering capacities.

The pregnant woman acquires approximately 7 l of extra water, comprising about 60 percent of the weight gain of pregnancy (Browne, 1973). Some 1,300 ml of this increased water load is contained in the plasma and 2,500 ml in the interstitial fluid. Much of this fluid acquisition is probably due to sodium retention in response to increased aldosterone secretion during pregnancy (Plentl and Gray, 1959; Davey et al., 1961).

Serum osmolarity decreases during pregnancy, reflecting in general a relative fall in concentration of serum electrolytes (Macdonald and Good, 1971; Robertson and Cheyne, 1972). The one notable exception is chloride, which undergoes a drop early in gestation and then rises to approximately nonpregnant values from midgestation to term (Macdonald *et al.*, 1973).

The literature on alterations in serum electrolytes during pregnancy is sparse. It is noteworthy that the figures given in current texts and handbooks (see for example *The Physiology of Human Pregnancy* by F. E. Hytten and I. Leitch, 1971, Blackwell; *Handbook of Obstetrical and Gynecological Data* by R. C. Goodlin, 1972, Geron-X, Inc.; and "Maternal and Fetal Blood Constituents" by T. H. Kirschbaum and J. C. DeHaven, in *Biology of Gestation*, vol. II, *The Fetus and Neonate*, N. S. Assali, ed., 1968, Academic Press) are all derived from Newman's (1957) study of only 27 women. The study did involve serial or longitudinal determinations on the same women throughout gestation, which tends to yield more useful data with less variability than cross-sectional studies. Similarly, a recent study of Macdonald *et al.* (1973) involved only five women, but, because all were induced to ovulate, preconception as well as early pregnancy values followed by closely timed samples throughout gestation make these data useful (Figure 3-1).

As can be noted in the tables, considerable interlaboratory variability is encountered, presumably reflecting methodologic differences. Various laboratories tend to standardize values internally, and there is little cross-standardization between laboratories or at a national level. Thus, in attempting to define normal values for electrolytes, a variety of mean values are encountered for each ion (Table 3-1). These problems make it important that sample bloods are obtained either prior to conception or postpartum from women whose alterations in serum electrolytes are being followed during pregnancy.

BICARBONATE

The pCO_2 begins to fall early in pregnancy in a manner suggesting an increased sensitivity of the respiratory centers, which may be induced by progesterone (Goodland *et al.*, 1953). The lowering of pCO_2 results in a reduction in plasma bicarbonate (Table 3-2; Figure 3-1) in order to maintain an appropriate pH level. It is noteworthy that unlike serum osmolality, sodium, or potassium, which show a nadir early in gestation with some recovery by term (although not to prepregnant levels), plasma CO_2 combining power continues its slow but steady decrease throughout gestation (Figure 3-1). It has been suggested (Hytten and Lind, 1973) that the drop in plasma bicarbonate may contribute to lowered sodium levels and, thus, osmolality.

Newman (1957) determined serum bicarbonate levels by means of

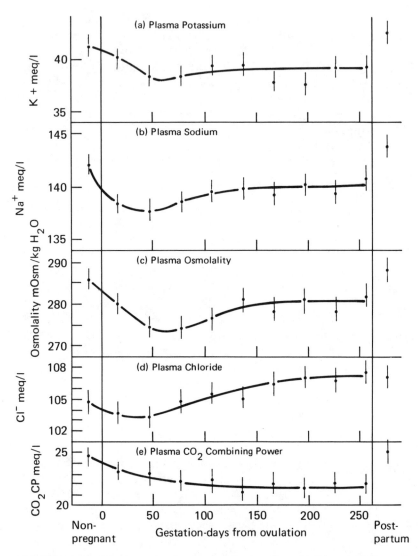

FIGURE 3-1 Serial changes in plasma potassium, sodium chloride, osmolality, and CO_2 combining power in moving from the nonpregnant state through pregnancy into the puerperium. The points denote mean values, and the vertical lines indicate ± 1 SD of the mean. K^+, Na^+, and CO_2CP values are derived from five individuals, while Cl^- values refer to three individuals only. From Macdonald et al. (1973).

TABLE 3-1   Electrolyte Levels in Normal Adults

References	Electrolyte	No.	Mean	95% Range
Schwab (1962)	Bicarbonate (meq/l)	15	24.9	21.3–28.5
Stutzman and Amatuzio (1952)	Calcium	48	5.09	4.7–5.5
Gyllensward and Josephson (1957)	(meq/l)	—	5.2	4.8–5.6
Bauditz (1967)		70	4.74	4.56–4.92
Schales and Schales (1953)	Chloride	100	102.7	99–110
Flear and Hughes (1963)	(meq/l)	157	106	101–111
Wallach *et al.* (1962)	Magnesium	77	2.0	1.70–2.30
Hanze (1962)	(meq/l)	46	1.70	1.30–2.10
Hanze (1962)		40	1.73	1.45–2.01
MacIntyre (1963)		76	1.66	1.50–1.82
Stewart *et al.* (1963)		100	1.74	1.52–1.96
Thiers (1965)		58	1.89	1.6–2.2
Basinski (1965)		97	1.80	1.28–2.32
Greenberg *et al.* (1960)	Phosphorus		3.5–4.0[a]	
Wertheim *et al.* (1954)	(mg%)		3.36	2.56–4.16
Flear and Hughes (1963)	Potassium	157	4.30	3.40–5.20
Marongiv *et al.* (1966)	(meq/l)	37	4.05	3.37–4.73
Funder and Wieth (1966)		22	4.4	3.6–5.2
Gessler (1961)	Sodium	20	144.5	138–151
Marongiv *et al.* (1966)	(meq/l)	37	143.1	136–151
Flear and Hughes (1963)		157	138	132–144
Bergström and Hultman (1962)		20	142.6	132–148
Marongiv *et al.* (1966)		106	138.4	132–145

[a]Read from regression curve for females, ages 20–40.

TABLE 3-2   Bicarbonate Levels (meq/l) during Pregnancy

References	No. Patients	Non-pregnant	Trimester 1	Trimester 2	Trimester 3
Newman (1957) (serum)	27	25.9 (22.0–30.0)	24.6 (22.0–27.0)	23.9 (21.5–26.5)	23.2 (20.5–26.0)
Hytten and Lind (1973) (plasma)	15,27,69,12	23.4	22.0	21.5	21.2
Brandstetter and Schuller (1959)[a] (serum)	10,20,20,30	26.4 (25.3–27.5)	24.5 (23.6–25.4)	22.8 (22.0–23.6)	22.8 (21.9–23.7)

[a]Cross-sectional study.

the titration method of Van Slyke. Following CO_2 estimations with Astruss apparatus, serum bicarbonate was also calculated in pregnancy (MacRae and Palarradji, 1967). Carbon dioxide combining power (Macdonald et al., 1973) was measured by Technicon (Figure 3-1) and yields results similar to those of direct bicarbonate determinations (Newman, 1957; Hytten and Lind, 1973).

No alterations in plasma bicarbonate have been found in conjunction with various complications of pregnancy (MacRae and Palarradji, 1967), even in conditions such as pneumonia or pneumonectomy, which would be expected to interfere with respiratory function.

CALCIUM

Alterations in serum calcium levels during pregnancy have received more study (Table 3-3) because of interest in direct hormonal regulation of calcium levels and because of disease states such as maternal hyperparathyroidism and neonatal hypocalcemia.

All investigators agree that total serum calcium levels decline during gestation (Table 3-3). A slight reprieve from this decline is encountered during the last few weeks before term (Michel, 1971). Investigators vary on the extent of the observed decrease; as can be seen in Table 3-3 it varies from approximately 2 to 10 percent less than prepregnant values.

Alterations in serum calcium level closely parallel the gradual decline in serum proteins occurring during pregnancy (Pitkin, 1975). If so, this would mean that only bound calcium would decrease during pregnancy, while ionic or free calcium stays constant. Indeed, diffusable calcium does not appear to change during pregnancy according to studies involving filtration (Andersch and Oberst, 1936), ultracentrifugation (Kerr et al., 1962), and calcium ion electrode determinations (Reitz et al., 1972). It should be noted, however, that Tan and colleagues (1972) (Table 3-3) have reported a decrease in ionized calcium during pregnancy. However, there are only two studies in the literature (Reitz et al., 1972; Tan et al., 1972) that involve calcium electrode analysis of serum ionic calcium since the instrumentation is new and notoriously tricky to use. Thus, more studies are needed in this area.

Serum levels of parathyroid hormone (PTH) increase during pregnancy (Reynolds et al., personal communication; Cushard et al., 1972; Reitz et al., 1972; Samaan et al., 1973). Determinations of plasma calcitonin (CT) levels in pregnancy are still ongoing. Samaan et al. (1973) have reported that the levels rise during gestation. Recently, Reynolds and co-workers (personal communication) have observed a

References	No. Patients	Nonpregnant	Trimester 1	Trimester 2	Trimester 3	% Decrease (Nonpregnant and 3d Trimester)
Total calcium						
Newman (1957)	27	4.86 (4.5–5.5)[a]	4.94 (4.45–5.55)	4.81 (4.1–5.5)	4.69 (4.15–5.05)	3.5
Reynolds et al. (personal communication)[b]	40, 33, 29, 33	4.6 (4.36–4.85)	4.84 (4.66–5.02)	4.62 (4.38–4.88)	4.52 (4.29–4.73)	1.7
Kerr et al. (1962)	24	5.2 (5.0–5.4)			4.7[c] (4.5–4.9)	9.6
Tan et al. (1972)[b]	15, 44, 61		4.40 (4.32–4.50)	4.47 (4.42–4.53)	4.38 (4.35–4.42)	
Brandstetter and Schuller (1959)[b]	10, 20, 20, 30	5.08 (4.83–5.33)	4.89 (4.58–5.20)	4.82 (4.53–5.11)	4.74 (4.55–4.93)	6.6
Michel (1971)	100	5.03	8 wk 5.00 (4.71–5.29); 12 wk 4.97 (4.67–5.27)	16 wk 4.85 (4.56–5.14); 20 wk 4.92 (4.63–5.21); 24 wk 4.73 (4.42–5.04)	28 wk 4.69 (4.42–4.96); 32 wk 4.55 (4.33–4.77); 36 wk 4.54 (4.25–4.83); 40 wk 4.61 (4.34–4.88)	8.6
Ultrafiltrable calcium						
Kerr et al. (1962)		2.8 (2.6–3.0)			2.6[c] (2.4–2.8)	7.1
Ionic calcium						
Tan et al. (1972)	16, 55, 59		4.43 ± 0.12[d]	4.41 ± 0.06[d]	4.21 ± 0.04[d]	

[a] Values in parentheses are 95 percent range.
[b] Cross-sectional study.
[c] Six to eight months of gestation.
[d] Mean ± SE.

23

decrease in serum CT in pregnancy, a finding more consonant with the documented elevation in PTH over the course of gestation. Estrogen and progesterone injections given to a nonpregnant woman failed to alter calcium metabolism (Heaney and Skillman, 1971). However, serum calcium levels are reduced in women consuming progestational contraceptives (Simpson and Dale, 1972).

About 30 g of calcium is accrued by the pregnant women, mostly during the last trimester (Pitkin, 1975), making calcium the electrolyte accumulated in greatest quantity during gestation. The miscible calcium pool increases by some 20 percent during pregnancy (Heaney and Skillman, 1971), while the pool turnover and bone mineral accretion rates increase gradually during pregnancy to double the nonpregnant values. Intestinal absorption of calcium is twice normal levels early in gestation and remains this way throughout gestation (Heaney and Skillman, 1971). Even so, if maternal consumption of calcium is less than 2 g per day, balance studies suggest that maternal stores of this ion will be depleted in order to supply fetal demands (Duggin et al., 1974).

Mull and Bill (1934) serially studied large numbers of patients and noted a significantly greater decrease in total serum calcium near term in the winter and spring than in pregnancies terminating in the summer and fall. This study was performed 40 yr ago, and well could reflect seasonal alterations in dietary patterns. Recently (Watney et al., 1971; Olatunbosun et al., 1975), it has been noted that West Indian and Nigerian women do not exhibit the lowered serum calcium levels in the third trimester characteristically found in European, American, and Asian women. These investigators suggest adequate sunlight exposure tends to maintain normal serum calcium levels in the West Indian and Nigerian women.

CHLORIDE

In contrast to the other electrolytes, chloride changes relatively little during pregnancy. A slight increase (Macdonald and Good, 1971; Macdonald et al., 1973) in chloride levels with increasing gestation has been reported (Table 3-4). In a closely timed study throughout gestation (Figure 3-1), Macdonald et al. (1973) observed an initial drop in plasma chloride, which recovered to prepregnant levels by the end of the first trimester and rose to a level some 2.5 percent above prepregnant levels at term.

Macdonald and Good (1972) suggest that steady or slightly increasing chloride levels are to be anticipated with gestation because plasma bicarbonate concentration decreases, which would shift chloride ions

TABLE 3-4 Chloride (meq/l) Levels during Pregnancy

References	No. Patients	Non-pregnant	Trimester		
			1	2	3
Newman (1957) (serum)	27	104.7 (100.5–109.5)	102.7 (98.7–107.0)	104.2 (96.0–107.6)	104.2 (98.0–108.0)
Brandstetter and Schuller (1959)[a] (serum)	10,20,20,30	105.3 (103.4–107.2)	104.2 (102.5–105.9)	103.9 (102.9–104.9)	102.5 (101.4–103.6)
Macdonald and Good (1971) (plasma)	204,191,210	—	101.2 ± 0.32	101.8 ± 0.31	102.0 ± 0.30

[a]Cross-sectional study.

out of cells into plasma and the extracellular fluid. The fact that the rise is so slight probably results from the diluting effect of increased plasma volume during pregnancy. It is noteworthy that primigravidae, who experience less increase in plasma volume than multigravidae, exhibit a greater increase in plasma chloride with advancing gestation (Macdonald and Good, 1972).

No studies seem to be available that correlate serum chloride measurements with complications of pregnancy.

The more recent studies (Macdonald and Good, 1971; Macdonald *et al.*, 1973) were performed by Technicon autoanalyzer; Newman (1957) used a titration method, as did Brandstetter and Schuller (1959). Thus, the disparity in the latter's data, where chloride reportedly decreased with gestation, cannot be explained methodologically. Greater reliance can probably be given to the studies of Macdonald (Macdonald and Good, 1971; Macdonald *et al.*, 1973) because of the greater numbers of patients involved and the conformity of their data.

MAGNESIUM

Although various workers do not report the same values, there is complete unanimity that this electrolyte decreases substantially as pregnancy proceeds (Table 3-5). The decreases reported over prepregnant values range from 7 to 12 percent. The decline would appear to reflect uncompensated dilution due to increasing plasma volume. In fact, if serum magnesium levels are corrected for hemodilution, pregnant women are hypomagnesic only during the first 120 days of gestation (DeJorge *et al.*, 1965).

PHOSPHORUS

After absorption, phosphorus enters the blood, wherein most of it circulates as orthophosphate ions. Proportionately (depending on pH), the concentrations of these ions are: $H_2PO_4^-$, 18.6; HPO_4^{2-}, 81.4; PO_4^{3-}, 0.008. Obviously, HPO_4^{2-} is the dominant phosphate ion in circulation. About 12 percent of plasma phosphorus is bound to proteins. Various investigators, utilizing different techniques, derived serum phosphate or inorganic phosphorus levels in measuring electrolytes during pregnancy. For comparative purposes, all values have been converted into serum inorganic phosphorus (Table 3-6). This is not altogether satisfactory because today most clinical laboratories measure serum HPO_4^{2-} levels in patients.

Some years ago, Mull and Bill (1934) serially determined inorganic

TABLE 3-5 Serum Magnesium (meq/l) Levels during Pregnancy

References	No. Patients	Non-pregnant	Trimester 1	Trimester 2	Trimester 3	% Decrease
Newman (1957)	27	1.67 (1.35–2.4)	1.57 (1.34–2.2)	1.53 (1.14–1.8)	1.47 (1.03–1.74)	12
Brandstetter and Schuller (1959)[a]	10,20,20,30	1.78 (1.50–2.06)	1.75 (1.57–1.93)	1.72 (1.49–1.95)	1.65 (1.51–1.79)	7
Michel (1971)	100	1.61	1.65 ± 0.17 8 wk 1.55 ± 0.22 12 wk	1.53 ± 0.23 16 wk 1.46 ± 0.28 20 wk 1.56 ± 0.26 24 wk	1.48 ± 0.17 28 wk 1.46 ± 0.21 32 wk 1.48 ± 0.20 36 wk 1.45 ± 0.20 40 wk	9
Reynolds et al. (personal communication)	33,29,29,37	—	1.51 (1.36–1.66)	1.42 (1.30–1.54)	1.39 (1.36–1.42)	8

[a]Cross-sectional study.

27

TABLE 3-6   Serum Inorganic Phosphorus (mg%) Levels
during Pregnancy

References	No. Patients	Non-pregnant	Trimester		
			1	2	3
Newman (1957)	27	3.04	3.02	2.76	2.82
		(1.71–4.03)	(2.17–4.03)	(1.86–3.57)	(2.02–4.03)
Kerr et al. (1962)	24	3.5			3.0
		(3.1–3.9)			(2.5–3.5)
Tan et al. (1972)[a]	16,51,60		3.83	3.91	3.56
			(3.67–3.99)	(3.78–4.04)	(3.46–3.66)
Reynolds et al. (personal communication)[a]	33,29,37		4.11	4.33	4.53
			(3.49–4.73)	(3.53–5.13)	(3.48–5.56)

[a]Cross-sectional study.

phosphorus levels in a large number of pregnant women (Figure 3-2).
Note the gradual fall in inorganic phosphorus, reaching a nadir at about
29 wk of gestation, followed by some recovery towards nonpregnant
values 1 to 2 wk before term. More recent studies yield confounding
data (Table 3-6). Three groups (Newman, 1957; Kerr et al., 1962; Tan
et al., 1972) observed a downward trend in phosphate (Newman, 1957)
or inorganic phosphorus (Kerr et al., 1962; Tan et al., 1972) toward
term. Two more recent studies (Reynolds et al., personal communication; Simpson and Dale, 1972), involving cross-sectional determinations, found elevated total serum phosphorus levels near the end of
gestation. All methods (Table 3-6, Figure 3-2) involved variations of
colorimetric procedures.

POTASSIUM

Blood levels of potassium appear to decrease throughout the first
two-thirds of pregnancy and rise slightly before term (Table 3-7, Figure
3-1). Interestingly, both the decrease and increase are statistically
significant in multigravidae but not in primigravidae (Macdonald and
Good, 1972). It is likely that hemodilution is responsible for the fall in
potassium early in gestation. The increase in serum potassium late in
gestation is harder to explain. Aldosterone influences on the distal
kidney tubule regulate the reabsorption of sodium but probably not
potassium in pregnancy (Ehrlich, 1971). A redistribution of extracellu-

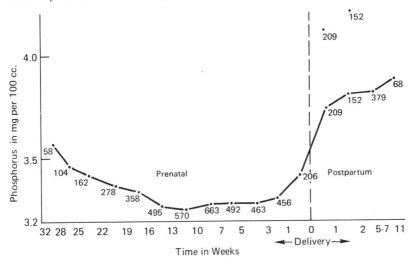

FIGURE 3-2   The curve illustrates the fall and recovery of the inorganic phosphorus of the serum during pregnancy, with the sharp increase following delivery. The numbers indicate the determinations made in each interval, the average of which is plotted. The two isolated points in the first and second weeks postpartum are values uncorrected for the effect of carbohydrate metabolism. No determinations were made from the end of the second to the beginning of wk 5 postpartum. From Mull and Bill (1934).

lar and intracellular potassium may occur; red blood cells tend to lose potassium in late pregnancy (Herbinger and Wichmann, 1967).

No correlations of alterations in serum potassium levels with pregnancy complications were found in the literature.

SODIUM

Plasma sodium levels decrease, probably beginning shortly after conception and continuing through wk 28 (Table 3-8). Only Newman (1957) reported increasing sodium levels throughout gestation. However, his values for the first trimester are lower than those for nonpregnant women, suggesting a decrease early in gestation. Some recovery in serum sodium towards the end of gestation has been noted (Macdonald and Good, 1971) (Figure 3-1). Again, multigravidae, who experience a greater expansion of plasma value than do primigravidae, exhibit the greater decrease in plasma sodium levels (Macdonald and Good, 1972). It has been suggested (Macdonald and Good, 1971) that the decrease in sodium early in gestation may be countered by the increasing production of aldosterone later in gestation. It is noteworthy, however, that

TABLE 3-7 Potassium (meq/l) Levels during Pregnancy

References	No. Patients	Non-pregnant	Trimester 1	Trimester 2	Trimester 3
Newman (1957) (serum)	27	4.25 (3.15–5.2)	4.07 (3.15–5.2)	4.00 (3.15–4.65)	3.97 (3.15–4.45)
Brandstetter an l Schuller (1959)[a] (serum)	10,20,20,30	4.23 (4.07–4.39)	4.25 (4.06–4.44)	4.24 (4.08–4.40)	4.11 (3.99–4.23)
Macdonald and Good (1972) (plasma)	60	4.26 ± 0.13	–	3.99 ± 0.12 20 wk 3.92 ± 0.12 24 wk	3.87 ± 0.12 28 wk 4.10 ± 0.15 32 wk 4.26 ± 0.13 36 wk 4.21 ± 0.17 40 wk
Macdonald and Good (1971) (plasma)	198,196,209	–	3.83 ± 0.02	3.78 ± 0.03	4.00 ± 0.04

[a]Cross-sectional study.

TABLE 3-8 Sodium (meq/l) Levels during Pregnancy

References	No. Patients	Non-pregnant	Trimester		
			1	2	3
Newman (1957) (serum)	27	143.3 (136.5–150.0)	138.9 (135.0–144.5)	139.1 (131.0–144.0)	139.5 (132.5–143.0)
Brandstetter and Schuller (1959)[a] (serum)	10,20,20,30	146.1 (144.3–147.9)	144.0 (142.3–145.7)	141.1 (139.3–142.9)	139.7 (137.9–141.5)
Herbinger and Wichmann (1967) (plasma)	60	138.7 ± 0.8	–	136.4 ± 0.36 20 wk 136.3 ± 1.34 24 wk	138.6 ± 1.05 28 wk 137.3 ± 0.88 32 wk 136.7 ± 0.98 36 wk 136.7 ± 1.30 40 wk
Macdonald and Good (1971) (plasma)	205,198,210	–	135.5 ± 0.4	134.6 ± 0.4	134.8 ± 0.4

[a]Cross-sectional study.

31

diminishing sodium levels do not appear to be the cause of the increasing rate of release of aldosterone in pregnancy (Landau and Lugibihl, 1961). The role of aldosterone in conserving sodium in the pregnant woman is emphasized by the fact that extensive natriuresis accompanies suppression of aldosterone secretion in pregnant women (Ehrlich, 1971).

Progesterone enhances renal excretion of sodium (Landau and Lugibihl, 1961) and thus may be in part responsible for the lowered values encountered throughout pregnancy.

All values reported for sodium (Table 3-8, Figure 3-1) were determined by flame photometer.

REFERENCES

Andersch, M., and F. W. Oberst. 1936. Filterable serum calcium in late pregnant and paturient women, and in the newborn. J. Clin. Invest. 15:131–133.

Basinski, D. H. 1965. Magnesium (titon yellow). Stand. Methods Clin. Chem. 5:137–142.

Bauditz, W. 1967. Der plasmacalciumwert beim menschen und seine altersabhängigkeit. Z. Gesamte Exp. Med. 142:9–21.

Bergström, J., and E. Hultman. 1962. Normal plasma-sodium values. Lancet. 1:1132–1133.

Brandstetter, F., and E. Schuller. 1959. Schrumelektrolyte Indergraviditat. Arch. Gynaekol. 193:420–421.

Browne, J. C. 1973. 24-Water and electrolyte balance in pregnancy. Obstet. Gynecol., 4th ed. pp. 497–504.

Cushard, W. G., M. A. Creditor, J. M. Canterbury, and E. Reiss. 1972. Physiologic hyperparathyroidism in pregnancy. J. Clin. Endocrinol. Metab. 34:767–771.

Davey, D. A., W. J. O'Sullivan, and J. C. Browne. 1961. Total exchangeable sodium in normal pregnancy and pre-eclampsia. Lancet 1:519–523.

DeJorge, F. B., D. Delascio, A. B. de Ulhoa Cintra, and M. L. Antunes. 1965. Magnesium concentration in the blood serum of normal pregnant women. Obstet. Gynecol. 25:253–254.

Duggin, G. G., N. E. Dale, R. C. Lyneham, R. A. Evens, D. J. Tiller. 1974. Calcium balance in pregnancy. Lancet 2:926–927.

Ehrlich, E. N. 1971. Heparinoid-induced inhibition of aldosterone secretion in pregnant women. Am. J. Obstet. Gynecol. 109:963–970.

Flear, C. T. G., and P. Hughes. 1963. Electrolyte content of extracellular fluid in health and in congestive heart failure. Br. Heart J. 25:166–172.

Funder, J., and J. O. Wieth. 1966. Potassium, sodium, and water in normal human red blood cells. Scand. J. Clin. Lab. Invest. 18:167–180.

Gessler, U. 1961. Intra-und extracelluläre Elektrolytveränderungen bei metabolischer Acidose. Untersuchungen an Erythrocyten. Klin. Wochenschr. 39:232–238.

Goodland, R. L., J. G. Reynolds, A. B. McCoord, and W. T. Pommerenke. 1953. Respiratory and electrolyte effects induced by estrogen and progesterone. Fertil. Steril. 4:300–317.

Greenberg, B. G., R. W. Winters, and J. B. Graham. 1960. The normal range of serum inorganic phosphorus and its utility as a discriminant in the diagnosis of congenital hypophosphatemia. J. Clin. Endocrinol. Metab. 20:364–379.

Gyllensward C., and B. Josephson. 1957. The development of the serum electrolyte concentration in normal infants and children. Scand. J. Clin. Lab. Invest. 9:21–28.

Hanze, S. 1962. Der Magnesiumstoffwechel. Thieme, Stuttgart.

Heaney, R. P., and T. G. Skillman. 1971. Calcium metabolism in normal human pregnancy. J. Clin. Endocrinol. Metab. 33:661–670.

Herbinger, V. W., and H. Wichmann. 1967. Die Extrazellulären und Intraerythrozytaren Electrolyte Während der Zweiten Schwangerschaftshälfte. Gynaecologia 163:1–13.

Hytten, F. E., and T. Lind. 1973. Diagnostic Indices in Pregnancy. Ciba-Geigy, Basel, Switzerland. 122 pp.

Kerr, C., H. I. Loken, M. B. Glendening, G. S. Gordon, and E. W. Page. 1962. Calcium and phosphorous dynamics in pregnancy. Am. J. Obstet. Gynecol. 83:2–8.

Landau, R. L., and K. Lugibihl. 1961. The catabolic and natriuretic effects of progesterone in man. Recent Prog. Horm. Res. 17:249–292.

Macdonald, H. N., and W. Good. 1971. Changes in plasma sodium, potassium and chloride concentrations in pregnancy and the puerperium, with plasma and serum osmolality. J. Obstet. Gynaecol. Br. Commonw. 78:798–803.

Macdonald, H. N., and W. Good. 1972. The effect of parity on plasma sodium, potassium chloride and osmolality levels during pregnancy. J. Obstet. Gynaecol. Br. Commonw. 79:441–449.

Macdonald, H. N., W. Good, K. W. Hancock. 1973. Biochemical changes in pregnancies following ovulation-induction therapy. J. Obstet. Gynaecol. Br. Commonw. 80:481–485.

MacIntyre, I. 1963. Magnesium metabolism. Sci. Basis Med. Annu. Rev. pp. 216–234.

MacRae, D. J., and Palarradji, S. R. N. 1967. Maternal acid-base changes in pregnancy. J. Obstet. Gynaecol. Br. Commonw. 74:11–16.

Marongiv, F., H. J. Holtmeier, and A. von Klein-Wisenberg. 1966. Zur Bestimmung des Mineralgehaltes in Erythrocyten. Klin. Wochenschr. 44:1405–1412.

Michel, C. F. 1971. Zeitschrift für Geburtshilfe und der Serum-Magnesium-Gehalt in der Schwangerschaft und Unter der Geburt im Vergleich zum Serum-Kalzium. Z. Geburtshilfe Gynaekol. 174:276–285.

Mull, J. W., and A. H. Bill. 1934. Variations in serum calcium and phosphorus during pregnancy. Am. J. Obstet. Gynecol. 27:510–517.

Newman, R. L. 1957. Serum electrolytes in pregnancy, parturition, and puerperium. Obstet. Gynecol. 10:51–55.

Olatunbosun, D. A., F. A. Adeniyi, and B. K. Adadevoh. 1975. Serum calcium, phosphorus and magnesium levels in pregnant and non-pregnant Nigerians. Br. J. Obstet. Gynaecol. 82:568–571.

Pitkin, R. M. 1975. Calcium metabolism in pregnancy: a review. Am. J. Obstet. Gynecol. 121:724–737.

Plentl, A. A., and M. J. Gray. 1959. Total body water, sodium space, and total exchangeable sodium in normal and toxemic pregnant women. Am. J. Obstet. Gynecol. 78:472–478.

Reitz, R. E., T. A. Daane, J. D. Woods, and R. L. Weinstein. 1972. Human parathyroid hormone (HPTH)-calcium interrelations in pregnancy and newborn infants. Fourth Int. Congr. Endocrinol. pp. 208–209.

Reynolds, W. A., R. M. Pitkin, G. Hargis, W. Kawahara, and G. A. Williams. Personal communication.

Robertson, E. G., and G. A. Cheyne. 1972. Plasma biochemistry in relation to odema of pregnancy. J. Obstet. Gynaecol. Br. Commonw. 79:769–776.

Samaan, N. A., C. S. Hill, Jr., J. R. Beceiro, and P. N. Schultz. 1973. Immunoreactive calcitonin in medullary carcinoma of the thyroid in maternal and cord serum. J. Lab. Clin. Med. 81:671–681.

Schales, O., and S. S. Schales. 1953. Chloride. Stand. Methods Clin. Chem. 1:37–42.

Schwab, M. 1962. Das Säure-Basen-Gleichgewicht im arteriellen Blut und Liquor cerebrospinalisbei Chronischer Niereninsuffizienz. Klin. Wochenschr. 40:765–772.

Simpson, G. R., and F. Dale. 1972. Serum levels of phosphorus, magnesium and calcium in women utilizing combination oral or long-acting injectable progestational contraceptives. Fertil. Steril. 23:326–330.

Stewart, W. K., F. Hutchinson, and L. W. Fleming. 1963. The estimation of magnesium in serum and urine by atomic absorption spectrophotometry. J. Lab. Clin. Med. 61:858–872.

Stutzman, F. L., and D. S. Amatuzio. 1952. A study of serum and spinal fluid calcium and magnesium in normal humans. Arch. Biochem. 39:271–275.

Tan, C. M., A. Raman, and T. A. Sinnathyray. 1972. Serum ionic calcium levels during pregnancy. J. Obstet. Gynaecol. Br. Commonw. 79:694–697.

Thiers, R. E. 1965. Magnesium (flourometric). Stand. Methods Clin. Chem. 5:131–136.

Wallach, S., L. N. Cahill, F. H. Rogan, and H. L. Jones. 1962. Plasma and erythrocyte magnesium in health and disease. J. Lab. Clin. Med. 59:195–210.

Watney, P. J. M., G. W. Chance, P. Scott, and J. M. Thomson. 1971. Maternal factors in neonatal hypocalcaemia: a study in three ethnic groups. Br. Med. J. 2:432–436.

Weir, R. J., J. J. Brown, R. Fraser, A. F. Lever, R. W. Logan, G. M. McIlwaine, J. J. Morton, J. I. S. Robertson, and M. Tree. 1975. Relationship between plasma renin, renin-substrate, angiotensin II, aldosterone and electrolytes in normal pregnancy. J. Clin. Endocrinol. Metab. 40:108–115.

Wertheim, A. R., G. H. Eurman, and H. J. Kalinsky. 1954. Changes in serum inorganic phosphorus during intravenous glucose tolerance tests: in patients with primary (essential) hypertension, other disease states, and in normal man. J. Clin. Invest. 33:565–571.

4

Carbohydrate and
Lipid Metabolism

ROBERT H. KNOPP, AGUSTIN MONTES,
and MARIA R. WARTH

INTRODUCTION

Metabolic studies in pregnancy usually focus on the problem of maternal diabetes. Several diagnostic criteria are presently available for this purpose. Apart from blood glucose levels, however, firm norms for the other parameters are wanting. For example, available measurements of insulin, glucagon, ketone bodies, and lipids can provide only a general idea of normality and abnormality. Furthermore, little attention has been given to metabolic disorders in pregnancy other than diabetes.

The orientation of this review is to present examples of metabolic studies performed in pregnancy. Differences in analytical technique are emphasized where they can reconcile differing results. Also, the rationale for performing each metabolic study is briefly explained. While an attempt has been made to be comprehensive, space precludes mention of all contributors to a topic.

GLUCOSE

Urinary Glucose

A method for accurately measuring urinary glucose has been developed recently by Lind and Hytten (1972) employing a coupled

35

KNOPP *et al.*

hexokinase glucose-6-phosphate dehydrogenase system. Earlier glu-cose oxidase methods, including enzyme-impregnated paper strips, appear to be inhibited by interfering substances such as ascorbic acid, giving levels that are falsely low in pregnancy and limiting their value for screening purposes. With this new methodology, Lind and Hytten (1972) find that urinary glucose excretion is increased roughly five-, seven-, and eight-fold in the first, second, and third trimesters, respec-tively. However, the variation is very great not only between individ-uals (see Table 4-1) but also between days for the same individual. The variation is so great that the authors did not calculate averages for the three trimesters. While we have made such a calculation, it is certainly not intended to gloss over the impressive variability that is implicit in the large standard deviation and wide range. Similar problems with variable urinary glycosuria were previously observed by Sutherland *et al.* (1970) and Soler and Malins (1971).

While the variation in glycosuria appears to have some basis in altered proximal tubular glucose reabsorption, the explanation for variation in tubular transport of glucose is still lacking (Davison and Hytten, 1975). The unpredictable changes in glycosuria place in ques-tion the value of urinary glucose screening in pregnancy, especially since the glucose-oxidase strips also correlate poorly with quantitative urinary glucose determination (Davison and Lovedale, 1974).

TABLE 4-1   Mean Urinary Glucose Excretion in the Three Trimesters[a]

| | Urinary Glucose (mg/24 h) | | | |
| | | Weeks Gestation | | |
	Nonpregnant[b]	10–12	14–26	38–40
No.	22	38	107	154
Mean	61.2	318	417	502
SD	20.2	366	791	1,021
SE	4.3	59	77	83
Range	30–97	44–1,565	33–4,890	9–9,832

[a]Data calculated from Lind and Hytten (1972). Glucose determined by a hexokinase, glucose-6-phosphate dehy-drogenase method. In this study 30 subjects were followed serially through gestation. As great variation was observed within, as well as between, individuals, the authors did not summarize their data, necessitating the arbitrary summary above.
[b]Nonpregnant subjects in this study are postpartum 6–8 wk.

Methods for Glucose Measurements in Blood

Table 4-2 reviews important issues on the measurement of glucose in blood. Capillary blood glucose is higher than venous blood glucose, especially after glucose administration. Capillary blood is often used by European workers, while plasma is generally used in the United States. As long as appropriate standards are used, analysis of blood from either source should be informative.

A failure to distinguish between glucose determined on whole blood and that determined on plasma can lead to serious confusion, as, for example, in the interpretation of the glucose tolerance test. Glucose measurements can be converted from one form to the other using the conversion factors given in Table 4-2. Glucose is often measured on plasma, because it is technically simpler and avoids the effect of differing hematocrits seen in whole-blood glucose measurements (Tables 4-2 and 4-3). It is perhaps surprising to discover that all of the standards defining normal and abnormal are expressed in terms of whole-blood glucose. One reason is that standards were set some years ago when glucose was determined only on whole blood. The standards have become so ingrained that there is little likelihood of change occurring soon. Other methodological considerations, including venipuncture technique and use of sample tubes containing sodium fluoride as a glycolytic inhibitor, are also important (Table 4-2).

Analytical methods most often encountered are the "true glucose" methods of Somogyi-Nelson, Hoffman, and glucose oxidase. The Somogyi-Nelson and automated Hoffman ferricyanide methods have given identical results in field testing (O'Sullivan and McDonald, 1966). The neocuproine method in use on Autoanalyzer SMA 6/60 and 12/60 systems runs slightly lower than the other reduction methods (Carey et al., 1974). Glucose oxidase yields results 3–10 percent lower than the automated ferricyanide method (Gochman and Schmitz, 1972; Carey et al., 1974) (Table 4-2). Glucose oxidase methods are under active study, and many laboratories with SMA systems are switching to enzyme systems because of their specificity (Gochman and Schmitz, 1972; Carey et al., 1974; Lott and Turner, 1975). The presence of NaF as a glycolytic inhibitor has interfered with the peroxidase oxygen acceptor of older glucose oxidase systems (ADA Committee on Statistics, 1969) but not in newer methods (Gochman and Schmitz, 1972; Carey et al., 1974; Lott and Turner, 1975).

With respect to the effect of hematocrit on whole-blood glucose, the lower the hematocrit, the higher the resulting glucose (Table 4-3). If, for example, a borderline abnormal glucose tolerance test were ob-

TABLE 4-2   Guide to Interpreting Glucose Measurements

I. *Venous versus capillary blood*

Venous blood glucose concentrations are lower than in capillary blood. The difference is exaggerated after a glucose load and may range from 8 to 61 mg/dl higher in capillary blood (Seltzer, 1970; Lind *et al.*, 1972).

II. *Whole blood versus plasma glucose*

Whole blood glucose levels are lower than in plasma owing to the fact that red cells do not contain as much water as plasma. Thus blood glucose levels are also hematocrit dependent (see Table 4-3). Assuming an average pregnancy hematocrit of 35 (Hytten and Leitch, 1971), glucose concentrations can be converted from one form to the other (Zalme and Knowles, 1965; O'Sullivan and Kantor, 1963).
  a. Plasma glucose to whole blood glucose: WB = P × 0.88.
  b. Whole blood glucose to plasma glucose: P = WB × 1.14.

III. *Blood collection*

Blood should be collected in tubes containing an anticoagulant and sodium fluoride (2 mg/ml of blood) as a glycolytic inhibitor. Without this precaution, glucose will decrease 10–20 mg/100 ml/h at room temperature (Cornblath and Schwartz, 1966).

IV. *Analytical methods*

Methods that measure "true glucose" are preferable to the older methods (Folin Wu, Folin Malmros, and Hagedorn Jenson) that react with non-glucose-reducing substances (Seltzer, 1970). "True glucose" methods include:
  a. Reduction methods (Seltzer, 1970)
    1. Somogyi-Nelson (manual)
    2. Ferricyanide method of Hoffman (autoanalyzer I)
    3. Neocuproine (autoanalyzer II including SMA 6/60 and 12/60)
  b. Enzyme methods (Seltzer, 1970)
    1. Glucose oxidase-peroxidase system linked to an oxygen acceptor color indicator
    2. Hexokinase

V. *Correlations of various methods*

The Somogyi-Nelson and ferricyanide methods have seen the widest use and give nearly identical results (Sunderman, Jr., and Sunderman, 1961; O'Sullivan and McDonald, 1966). The neocuproine method is a few percent lower (Carey *et al.*, 1974). The glucose oxidase method may run 2 to 9 percent below Somogyi-Nelson (Sunderman, Jr., and Sunderman, 1961; Mager and Farese, 1965) and 3 to 10 percent below the ferricyanide method (Gochman and Schmitz, 1972; Carey *et al.*, 1974). Depending on the indicator, glucose oxidase measurements may yield falsely low values due to interference by other oxygen acceptors such as ascorbic acid and uric acid (Romano, 1973; Carey *et al.*, 1974; Lott and Turner, 1975).

TABLE 4-3 Ratios for Converting Glucose Concentrations in Plasma to Whole Blood at Various Hematocrits[a]

Hematocrit (%)	Ratio	Blood Glucose if Plasma Glucose = 200 (mg/dl)[b]
20	0.910	182.0
25	0.901	180.2
30	0.892	178.4
35	0.883	176.6
40	0.874	174.8
45	0.865	173.0
50	0.856	171.2

[a]Based on the formula of Zalme and Knowles (1965).
[b]Whole blood glucose = 13.2 + 0.88 × plasma glucose − 0.36 × Hct. At a hematocrit (Hct) of 36 (the average of 105 subjects) the conversion ratio is 0.88, which is that recommended by O'Sullivan and Kantor (1963) (see Table 4-2) and corresponds reasonably closely to the third-trimester hematocrit (Hytten and Leitch, 1971).

tained in a woman with a hematocrit of 25, she might be normal if her hematocrit were corrected to 35. A blood glucose value in this instance could be corrected by multiplying the glucose value by the ratio of 0.883/0.901. While such a correction may not be necessary very often, it does serve to illustrate the extent of the hematocrit effect on whole-blood glucose.

Fasting Glucose in Pregnancy

After an overnight fast, plasma glucose is reduced in pregnancy. The reduction is gradual but is noted consistently in the first trimester and progresses as term approaches. The condition is independent of the method of glucose measurement, having been first observed in whole blood by Silverstone *et al.* (1961) (Table 4-4) and confirmed by O'Sullivan (1970) (see Table 4-7) but also seen in capillary blood (see Table 4-6) and plasma (see Tables 4-9, 4-13, 4-16, and 4-20). While glucose utilization by the growing fetus contributes to this finding in late gestation (Freinkel, 1965), it seems less likely in early gestation when the conceptus is small, implying other regulatory factors.

Postprandial Glucose

Table 4-5 presents mean and two standard deviations above the mean for glucose levels in third-trimester subjects who had eaten breakfast at an earlier specified time. These data were obtained from ambulatory

TABLE 4-4   Fasting Whole Blood Glucose at Various Stages in Pregnancy[a]

	Blood Glucose (mg/dl)[b]				
	Non-pregnant	Trimester			1 wk Post-partum
		1	2	3	
No.[c]	30	21	20	20	25
Mean[d]	65.9	61.3	59.1	59.6	56.1
SE	1.2	1.5	1.6	1.9	2.0
Range	52–84	50–75	45–77	44–78	40–91

[a]Data of Silverstone *et al.* (1961).
[b]Somogyi-Nelson method.
[c]All subjects were selected to be free of diabetes.
[d]Similar fasting data are presented for venous whole blood (Table 4-7), capillary whole blood (Table 4-6), and plasma glucose (Tables 4-9, 4-13, 4-16, and 4-20).

pregnant subjects and are appropriately applied to a morning clinic setting (O'Sullivan *et al.*, 1966), inasmuch as the degree of postprandial hyperglycemia is not necessarily the same at the different meal times (Gillmer *et al.*, 1975; Persson and Lunell, 1975). These standards for postprandial glucose have the additional recommendation of having been "field tested" in a study of insulin therapy in gestational diabetes (O'Sullivan *et al.*, 1974a). Specifically, when the postprandial glucose in the third trimester exceeded the two SD limits, the insulin dosage was raised a minimum of 5 units (O'Sullivan *et al.*, 1974a). In our experi-

TABLE 4-5   Postbreakfast Blood Glucose in Third-Trimester Nondiabetic Ambulatory Subjects[a]

Time after Initiation of Breakfast (h)	No.	Blood Glucose (mg/dl)[b]	
		Mean ± SD	2 SD above Mean
½–1	54	81.6 ± 16.4	114.4
1–2	323	74.3 ± 15.2	104.7
2–3	166	68.6 ± 12.6	93.8
3–4	54	67.3 ± 12.5	92.3
<4 or fasting	77	65.9 ± 9.3	84.1

[a]Data of O'Sullivan *et al.* (1966). Diets consisted of 30 cal/kg of ideal body weight with 1.5–2.0 g/kg of protein, and 40 per cent of calories as fat. The amount taken at breakfast is unspecified.
[b]Somogyi-Nelson method.

ence, this procedure has proved to be safe and efficient and minimizes delays in "keeping up" with a rising glucose in late gestation.

Postprandial glucose measurements using capillary whole blood have been reported by Victor (1974) on hospitalized subjects (Table 4-6). It is interesting that the 12 M. and 7 P.M. mean values are higher in the third trimester than in the O'Sullivan study (Table 4-5) despite the fact that the measurements were made with glucose oxidase (Table 4-6), which should give lower values than the Somogyi-Nelson method. Presumably the higher values observed by Victor are due to the tendency of capillary glucose to be higher than venous whole blood, particularly in the postprandial state (Table 4-2). The fact that these measurements were obtained in hospitalized subjects who had reduced activity and illnesses (albeit nondiabetic) that necessitated admission could also be a factor in the higher values (Victor, 1974). The sensible use of these values would be the hospital setting at the times specified if capillary whole blood is used. Conversion of capillary blood glucose to venous blood glucose in pregnancy has been tried, but it is not considered to be reliable (Lind *et al.*, 1972).

Another screening method is the 1-h glucose measurement following ingestion of 50 g of oral glucose (O'Sullivan *et al.*, 1973). As described by O'Sullivan *et al.* (1973), this test was used in an afternoon prenatal registration clinic regardless of the time or amount of lunch previously consumed. A whole-blood glucose at 1 h of greater than 130 mg/dl proved to be a better predictor of abnormal glucose tolerance in

TABLE 4-6   Fasting and Postprandial Glucose at Various Times in Gestation in Nondiabetic Hospitalized Subjects[a]

Gestation (wk)	No.	Time (h pc) 7 A.M. (12.5)	No.	Time (h pc) 12 M. (0.75)	3 P.M. (3.75)	7 P.M. (0.50)
Nonpregnant	180	78 ± 11[b]	45	114 ± 22	92 ± 18	108 ± 18
5–20	88	73 ± 9[c]	35	103 ± 23	88 ± 25	98 ± 21
21–32	85	70 ± 9[d]	39	105 ± 17	82 ± 14	95 ± 21
33–36	83	67 ± 8	33	104 ± 22	80 ± 15	95 ± 21
37–38	46	66 ± 8	29	92 ± 17	79 ± 10	86 ± 15
39–	102	65 ± 9	80	91 ± 16	76 ± 13	86 ± 15

[a]Data of Victor (1974). Hospital diet consisted of 2,200 kcal and 246 g of carbohydrate daily; amount given at breakfast not specified. Capillary whole blood was measured by a glucose oxidose autoanalyzer method.
[b]Mean ± SD. Each value is compared statistically to that immediately preceding it.
[c]$P < 0.001$.
[d]$P < 0.01$.

pregnancy than a number of clinical criteria, including poor obstetrical history, a previous baby weighing greater than 9 lb, maternal obesity, and family history of diabetes (O'Sullivan *et al.*, 1973).

Oral Glucose Tolerance

For many years it was debated that there was no effect of pregnancy on oral glucose tolerance (Jackson, 1965) or, if differences did exist, delays in glucose absorption and other possible variables invalidated interpretation (Burt, 1960a). The first objection is answered by Tables 4-7, 4-8, and 4-9, where there is a clear elevation in glucose in late gestation after oral glucose challenge. With the 50-g dose (Table 4-9), the challenge to homeostasis is less and the glucose elevation is perhaps more subtle. The shift to hyperglycemia in the later portion of the test is particularly noteworthy (Table 4-9).

The question of interpretation was at one time confounded by the application to pregnancy of a variety of standards derived for nonpregnant individuals. O'Sullivan and Mahan (1964) resolved the problem by deriving standards specific to pregnancy itself (Table 4-8). Apart from the fact that there is security in large numbers of test subjects (Table 4-8), this study has the added advantage that the subjects were randomly selected and are therefore representative of mothers attending the two hospital clinics involved. Whether or not these data can be applied to other populations differing in socioeconomic, dietary, and racial background is yet to be determined. To date, there is no evidence to support these possibilities. In any case, the O'Sullivan criteria are the most scientifically obtained criteria for interpreting the oral glucose tolerance in pregnancy. Notice in Table 4-8 that the criteria are derived

TABLE 4-7   Effect of Pregnancy on 100-g Oral Glucose Tolerance in 163 Subjects Studied Pre- and Postpartum[a]

| | Whole-Blood Glucose (mg/dl)[b] at: | | | |
	0 h	1 h	2 h	3 h
Average 31 wk gestation[c]	69.1 ± 10.4	111.8 ± 27.3	94.4 ± 24.3	81.5 ± 20.8
Postpartum[d]	75.9 ± 12.7	87.7 ± 22.7	80.5 ± 17.4	73.1 ± 17.0

[a]From O'Sullivan *et al.* (1970).
[b]Hoffman autoanalyzer method.
[c]Mean age 25.5 yr; all subjects previously screened negative for diabetes.
[d]All differences between pregnant and postpartum are statistically significant.

TABLE 4-8 Tolerance to 100-g Oral Glucose in 752 Randomly Selected Pregnant Subjects[a]

A. *Characteristics of Subjects Studied*

Median age	24 (range, 13–44)
Median parity	2 (range, 0–9)
Race	60% Caucasian, 40% Negro
No. in each trimester	
1st	20
2d	339
3d	393
Dietary preparation	250 g carbohydrate for 3 days

B. *Results*

	Whole-Blood Glucose (mg/dl)[b] at:			
	0 h	1 h	2 h	3 h
Mean ± SD	69.3 ± 10.4	103.6 ± 30.8	91.7 ± 25.8	79.4 ± 24
2 SD upper limit	90	165	143	127
O'Sullivan criteria[c]				
Whole blood	90	165	145	125
Plasma[d]	103	188	165	143

[a]From O'Sullivan and Mahan (1964).
[b]Somogyi-Nelson methodology.
[c]Two or more elevated values constitute an abnormal test.
[d]Plasma criteria are calculated from whole blood × 1.14.

from a group about evenly divided between second and third trimester. While possible diagnostic distinctions between second and third trimesters are not provided, standards applicable to the transition period between second and third trimester have practical value, since most women register around this time; diabetes is most likely to become manifest at 26–28 wk gestation (Pedersen, 1967), and insulin treatment should be instituted at this time to be beneficial (O'Sullivan *et al.*, 1974a).

The fact that glucose tolerance deteriorates as gestation proceeds is illustrated in Table 4-10, which for practical purposes compares glucose tolerance tests done in the second and third trimesters (Wilkerson and O'Sullivan, 1963). These data illustrate that diagnostic criteria specific to each trimester are still needed.

The data shown in Table 4-11 are the result of studies to determine

TABLE 4-9 Tolerance to 50-g Oral Glucose at Various Times in Gestation in 19 Healthy Subjects[a]

Gestational Age	Plasma Glucose (mg/dl)[b] at:							
	0 min	15 min	30 min	45 min	60 min	75 min	90 min	120 min
Nonpregnant[c]	79.8 ± 5.7[d]	109.8 ± 11.7	114.8 ± 19.3	109.0 ± 22.5	91.1 ± 21.4	85.1 ± 20.5	82.5 ± 16.7	77.4 ± 19.7
10 wk	75.0 ± 8.3	104.9 ± 14.9	112.3 ± 21.5	111.9 ± 24.0	100.2 ± 26.7	93.7 ± 18.9	89.4 ± 22.6	87.1 ± 23.0
20 wk	71.1 ± 7.2	95.4 ± 11.4	105.5 ± 18.9	107.1 ± 23.8	99.2 ± 23.0	93.0 ± 20.7	83.5 ± 23.6	70.8 ± 17.5
30 wk[e]	74.3 ± 7.2	101.3 ± 16.0	119.1 ± 23.4	122.3 ± 28.8	111.7 ± 24.2	101.2 ± 22.8	96.6 ± 22.2	79.1 ± 17.0
38 wk[f]	68.8 ± 7.7	89.7 ± 12.8	113.1 ± 15.5	121.7 ± 20.7	121.5 ± 19.7	111.3 ± 20.9	102.5 ± 19.9	81.3 ± 18.3

[a]From Lind et al. (1973).
[b]Glucose determined with glucose oxidase-peroxidose system.
[c]Nonpregnant subjects were the previously pregnant subjects 10–12 wk postpartum; only one was lactating.
[d]Mean ± SD.
[e]Mean maximal increment significantly greater than nonpregnant (P < 0.01).
[f]Mean maximal increment significantly greater than nonpregnant (P < 0.001).

TABLE 4-10 Comparison of Glucose Tolerance Tests Performed in Two Successive Trimesters[a]

Test	Glucose (mg/dl)[b] at:			
	0 h	1 h	2 h	3 h
First Trimester	69.4	94.9	85.3	73.9
Second Trimester	69.8	111.5	93.3	82.5
Difference	0.4 ± 0.8^c	16.6 ± 1.9^d	8.0 ± 1.5^d	8.6 ± 1.5^d

[a]Data of Wilkerson and O'Sullivan (1963). With seven exceptions, the comparison is between the second and third trimesters.
[b]Somogyi-Nelson method.
[c]Mean ± SE.
[d]Difference is significantly different from 0 ($P < 0.001$ in all instances).

the effect of age and increasing parity on the oral glucose tolerance test (OGTT). Glucose tolerance tests were performed in three successive pregnancies in 52 third-trimester subjects (O'Sullivan and Mahan, 1966). Little effect of age over this 4-yr span can be clearly detected. However, even if OGTT standards should rise with age, the range of expectant mothers is fairly narrow, and, even if older gravidas might be slightly over-diagnosed, it appears permissible since the >25-yr-old group is at greatest risk of neonatal losses in gestational diabetes (O'Sullivan *et al.*, 1974a).

Different doses of glucose and methods of glucose determination require their own specific standards. Guttorm (1974) has obtained such standards (Table 4-12) using capillary blood and measuring glucose with glucose oxidase. Characteristically, the postglucose standards are

TABLE 4-11 Effect of Age on Repeat Glucose Tolerance Tests in 52 Third-Trimester Subjects[a]

Observed Pregnancy	Age	Glucose (mg/dl)[b] at:			
		0 h	1 h	2 h	3 h
1	23.5	69.9 ± 9.6^c	108.8 ± 28.1	91.7 ± 27.6	81.0 ± 17.2
2	25.6	73.7 ± 8.3	105.9 ± 24.8	91.4 ± 17.6	81.5 ± 17.7
3	27.4	75.7 ± 8.7	110.9 ± 21.4	95.4 ± 17.5	81.8 ± 19.1

[a]Based on O'Sullivan and Mahan (1966).
[b]Hoffman autoanalyzer method.
[c]Mean ± SD.

TABLE 4-12 Upper Limits (2 SD) to Oral Glucose (1 g/kg) in 154 Pregnant Subjects Screening Negative for Possible Diabetes[a]

	2 SD Upper Limit for Glucose (mg/dl)[b] at:							
	0 min	30 min	45 min	60 min	90 min	120 min	150 min	180 min
Plasma	103	200	228	227	197	167	148	130
Whole blood	86	168	191	190	165	140	121	109

[a]From Guttorm (1974).
[b]Glucose measured on capillary blood with a glucose oxidase method.

higher with capillary blood despite the lower glucose dose (70 g per 70 kg of body weight) and use of the glucose oxidase method.

Objective criteria for the 50-g OGTT are hard to find. They might be found in the Lind et al. (1973) data (Table 4-9), but the number of subjects is small. Criteria of the WHO Expert Committee (1965) discussed in Hytten and Lind's monograph (1973) are inexact and are not specific to pregnancy.

Recently, the H test has been devised for interpreting the shape of the pregnancy GTT (Billewicz et al., 1973). Interestingly, Lind et al. (1973) find that the shape of the curve changes as gestation proceeds, while Gillmer et al. (1975) do not. Further work is required to establish the usefulness of this analytical technique.

Intravenous Glucose Tolerance Tests

Another way of meeting objections to the oral GTT is to administer the glucose dose intravenously and circumvent possible effects of delayed glucose absorption. Again the parallel debate has arisen over whether the intravenous glucose tolerance test (IVGTT) in pregnant subjects is greater (Silverstone et al., 1961), the same (Bleicher et al., 1964; Yen et al., 1971), or less (Picard et al., 1968; O'Sullivan et al., 1970; Edstrom et al., 1974) than in nonpregnant ones. While a detailed review of this question can be found elsewhere (O'Sullivan et al., 1975), examining the glucose values of IVGTTs done in the third trimester and after 6 wk postpartum discloses differences (Table 4-13). Specifically, glucose values antepartum are lower in the early portion of the test.

For calculation of the fractional rate of glucose disappearance (k) in the IVGTT (Table 4-14), data are transformed to logarithms or plotted on semilog paper to obtain an approximate straight line function. A greater

TABLE 4-13   Mean Blood Glucose Values in the 25-g Intravenous Glucose Tolerance Test in 149 Subjects[a]

Time (min)	Blood Glucose (mg/dl)[b]		
	Antepartum[c]	Postpartum	Difference
0	77[d]	82	−4.7[e]
5	263	286	−24.2[e]
10	213	234	−20.7[e]
20	169	175	−5.1
30	137	137	0.8
40	116	114	1.4
50	100	100	0.9
60	88	90	−2.2

[a]From O'Sullivan and Mahan (1964).
[b]Glucose method: autoanalyzer ferricyanide.
[c]Mean gestational age was 30 wk.
[d]Results reported by Silverstone *et al.* (1961) are systematically lower by about 15–20 mg/dl (Somogyi-Nelson method). Results for a 37.5-dose in 77 subjects are (mg/dl): (5) 349, (10) 273, (20) 212, (30) 169, (40) 137, (50) 114, (60) 98 (O'Sullivan *et al.*, 1974b).
[e]Differences significant at $P < 0.01$.

curvilinearity persists in the postpartum data compared to antepartum (O'Sullivan *et al.*, 1970). In addition, O'Sullivan *et al.* (1970) have found varied degrees of nonlinearity among individual antepartum and postpartum tests. For these reasons, these authors have developed rules to truncate individual curves to use only the most linear portion for calculating k. Previous workers always used the same portions of the IVGTT curve in comparing pregnant and nonpregnant subjects (Silverstone *et al.*, 1961; Bleicher *et al.*, 1964; Picard *et al.*, 1968; Yen *et al.*, 1971; Edstrom *et al.*, 1974) although the portion of the curve used differed between studies.

Three groups have now reported on the IVGTT in pregnancy using the truncation rules (O'Sullivan *et al.*, 1970; Yen *et al.*, 1971; Sutherland and Stowers, 1975).* In the two studies presenting postpartum com-

*Truncation rules of O'Sullivan *et al.* (1970):

(a) If there is evidence of incomplete mixing at 10 min as defined by a 10 min value 50 gm/100 ml higher than expected from the slope of the subsequent values, the 20-min value is the first one used in the calculation.

(b) If the whole-blood glucose concentration returns to the fasting region (100 mg/100 ml) prior to 60 min, the first value below 100 mg/100 ml is the end point in the calculation.

(c) If there is a leveling of the slope (two successive values < 5 mg/100-ml difference) prior to the return to the fasting region, the first of these two values is the end point for calculation.

TABLE 4-14 Intravenous Glucose Tolerance in Pregnancy (25-g Dose) Based on Actual Glucose Values[a]

| | | k (%/min) | | | | | |
| | | Trimester | | | Postpartum | | Non-pregnant |
References	No. Subjects	1	2	3	1 wk	6 wk	
Normal values							
Silverstone et al. (1961)	20–31[b]	2.42 ± 0.14[c]	1.92 ± 0.09	1.91 ± 0.10	1.58 ± 0.08	–	1.67 ± 0.08
Bleicher et al. (1964)	10	–	–	1.41 ± 0.09[c]	–	1.29 ± 0.12	–
Billis and Rastogi (1966)	5 + 50	–	2.51 ± 0.56[d]	1.73 ± 0.33	–	–	–
Picard et al. (1968)	9	3.1	–	1.5	–	–	2.9
O'Sullivan et al. (1970)[e]	162–232	–	–	2.02 ± 0.05[c]	–	2.53 ± 0.10	–
Sutherland and Stowers (1975)	11	3.64 ± 1.01[d]	2.79 ± 0.75	1.93 ± 0.16	–	–	–
Yen et al. (1971)	10	–	–	1.69 ± 0.13[c]	–	1.88 ± 0.17	–
Edstrom et al. (1974)	12–14	2.51 ± 0.83[d]	2.41 ± 0.75	1.96 ± 0.76	–	–	2.17 ± 0.85
Lower limits							
Silverstone et al. (1961)	2 SD (lower limit)	1.37	1.18	1.13	0.93	–	–
Billis and Rastogi (1966)	2 SD (lower limit)	–	–	1.17	–	–	–
O'Sullivan et al. (1970)	Lower 5th percentile[f]	–	–	1.13	–	–	–

[a] The fractional turnover rate or k rate is calculated by visual fit on semilog paper (Silverstone et al., 1961) or by the method of least squares using the equation $BS = BS_n e^{k'}$ where BS_t = blood glucose at any time, BS_0 = blood glucose at time zero, and k = rate of glucose fall with time (O'Sullivan et al., 1970). A reduced version of this equation is $69.3/t$, where t is the time for the log-transformed values for glucose to decrease by ½. O'Sullivan et al. (1970), Sutherland and Stowers (1975), and Yen et al. (1971) excluded non-log linear portions of the curve according to certain rules (see text). Nonlinearity was particularly striking in the postpartum tests.
[b] Subjects represent differing populations. All were prescreened to be nondiabetic except those of O'Sullivan et al. (1970), who were a randomly selected population attending a city hospital.
[c] Mean ± SE.
[d] Mean ± SD.
[e] In a separate study, O'Sullivan et al. (1974b) found that a 37.5-g glucose load produced a significantly greater k rate of 2.24 in 77 subjects ($P < 0.01$).
[f] Lower limits cannot be calculated directly from the SD since IV GTT data are skewed positively; log transformation served to normalize the data (O'Sullivan et al., 1970).

parisons (O'Sullivan *et al.*, 1970; Yen *et al.*, 1971) (Table 4-14) a lower *k* value is obtained in third-trimester subjects compared to postpartum. These results differ from the earlier studies of Silverstone *et al.* (1961) and Bleicher *et al.* (1964) in which the third-trimester results were slightly higher compared to those of nonpregnant controls (Table 4-14). While use of truncation rules may account for the differences, others (Picard *et al.*, 1968; Edstrom *et al.*, 1974) have found a lower third-trimester *k* value without these rules. Comparing the studies, the greatest variation is seen in the postpartum data, with the third-trimester data being surprisingly close. Differences in postpartum data may be due to the greater curvilinearity of the IVGTT curve postpartum and a differential effect of the truncation rules between the pre- and postpartum periods, as well as subject selection, timing of the postpartum test, and other methodological differences.

In contrast to the controversy over third-trimester and postpartum IVGTTs, some obvious consistencies are seen in Table 4-14 regardless of source or method of calculation. In every study there is an increase in the *k* value early in gestation and a progression downward as gestation proceeds. While the mechanism is not completely clear, an increased rate of glucose disposal could help explain the lower fasting glucose in early gestation (Table 4-4). The other consistent feature in these data is the agreement on the lower limit of normal in the third trimester in the three studies in which it has been assessed (Table 4-14). The conclusion is that Silverstone's original lower limit for *k* of 1.13 appears to be quite serviceable (Silverstone *et al.*, 1961).

More recently, Sutherland and Stowers (1975) and O'Sullivan *et al.* (1974b) have calculated *k* values based on the glucose increment over a specified baseline (Table 4-15). This is the method proposed initially by Amatuzio *et al.* (1953). Since none of the studies of this method in pregnancy report paired studies at greater than 6 wk postpartum, only Amatuzio's (1953) mean value serves as a comparison (Table 4-15). Again, the issue of the effect in late gestation versus postpartum is unresolved. However, the elevation in the first trimester followed by a decline is again seen in the data of Sutherland and Stower (1975). This method has the advantage that the *k* values are independent of the dose (confirming Amatuzio *et al.*, 1953) and also of body weight (O'Sullivan *et al.*, 1974b).

Special Studies: Responses to Insulin, Tolbutamide, Glucagon, and Arginine

The resistance to the hypoglycemic effect of intravenously administered insulin (Burt, 1956) was the first objective evidence of insulin

TABLE 4-15 Intravenous Glucose Tolerance Test in Pregnancy Based on Glucose Elevations above Specified Baseline Glucose[a]

References	Dose (g)	No.	Non-pregnant	k (%/min)		
				Trimester		
				1	2	3
Sutherland and Stowers (1975)	25	11	–	6.29 ± 1.26[b]	5.09 ± 1.01	3.64 ± 0.42[c]
O'Sullivan et al. (1974b)	25	232	–	–	–	5.20 ± 0.98[d]
O'Sullivan et al. (1974b)	37.5	77	–	–	–	5.00 ± 1.20[d]
Amatuzio et al. (1953)	25	40	3.61 (3.00–4.84)[e]	–	–	–

[a]The arbitrary baseline was the fasting glucose level in the hands of Sutherland and Stowers (1975) and of Amatuzio et al. (1953). O'Sullivan et al. (1975) plotted the increment above a level lower than fasting, which was estimated for each subject. Glucose measurements were on capillary blood with glucose oxidase (Sutherland and Stowers, 1975; wholeblood autoanalyzer ferricyanide (O'Sullivan et al., 1974b), and whole-blood Folin-Malmros (Amatuzio et al., 1953).

[b]All values are means ± SD.

[c]In the third trimester, Sutherland and Stowers (1975) used the lower limit of 2.97 of Amatuzio et al. (1953).

[d]There is no significant difference in k rate between the two doses.

[e]Range of values.

50

resistance in normal pregnancy (it had been recognized in diabetic pregnancy for many years [Skipper, 1933]) (Table 4-16). A similar impairment is seen in response to endogenous insulin in the intravenous tolbutamide test (Burt, 1958; Kalkhoff *et al.*, 1964; Spellacy *et al.*, 1965c) (Table 4-16).

The response to intravenous glucagon in the third trimester of pregnancy is not impaired, and in fact glucose levels are higher later in the test (Burt, 1957) (Table 4-16). The implication is that glucagon responsiveness is at least intact and that the elevated glucose levels may reflect diminished utilization of glucose. The glycemic response to arginine (Table 4-16) is of interest since it reflects in part arginine-stimulated glucagon release, which stimulates hepatic glycogenolysis, as arginine is not itself a gluconeogenic substrate. In the third trimester, the glucose rise is equal to or greater than the nonpregnant response. However, in the first and second trimesters, the glycemic response is lower. These results depend on a complex interplay between the plasma arginine level, which is reduced in late gestation (King *et al.*, 1971), glucose removal, which is increased early in gestation and then declines (Table 4-14), and the glycogenolytic-gluconeogenic stimulus, which is also altered as judged by basal insulin and glucagon levels (see Table 4-20). It is difficult to predict the precise role of glucagon from these data, and further studies are required.

INSULIN SECRETION IN PREGNANCY

Fasting Insulin

Basal insulin levels at various stages of gestation are presented in Tables 4-17 through 4-20. A significant elevation in basal insulin in the third trimester is seen in the data of Spellacy and Goetz (1963), Spellacy *et al.* (1965a, 1965b), and Bleicher *et al.* (1964) (Table 4-18) and Freinkel *et al.* (1975) and Kühl and Holst (1976) (Table 4-20). Basal insulin levels are significantly lower in the first and second trimesters compared to control (Tyson *et al.*, 1969) and compared to third trimester (Lind *et al.*, 1973). The data of Felig and Lynch (1970) in second-trimester subjects support these findings ($\bar{x} \pm$ SE): nonpregnant (6), 11.1 ± 1.1 μU/ml; pregnant (12) 6.5 ± 0.6 μU/ml ($P < 0.05$). The lower basal insulin levels in early and midgestation resemble the changes seen on high carbohydrate feeding of normal and mildly diabetic subjects (Brunzell *et al.*, 1971) and are consistent with an enhanced postglucose insulin response in the first and second trimesters (see below).

TABLE 4-16 Special Studies: Glucose Response in Pregnancy to Intravenous Insulin, Tolbutamide, Glucagon, and Arginine[a]

Study	No.	Glucose (mg/dl)[b] at:							
		0 min	10 min	20 min	30 min	40 min	50 min	60 min	90–120 min
Insulin (0.1 μ/kg)									
Nonpregnant	20	—	—	31.0 ± 7.8[c]	—	—	—	—	—
8–26 wk	20	—	—	34.6 ± 9.5	—	—	—	—	—
36–40 wk	20	—	—	57.6 ± 13.4	—	—	—	—	—
Tolbutamide (1 g/kg)									(120 min)
Nonpregnant	12	90.7 ± 2.2[c]	74.9 ± 4.6	—	57.5 ± 4.3	—	—	67.6 ± 1.4	77.7 ± 2.0
36–40 wk	12	84.0 ± 2.2	81.6 ± 2.3	—	72.1 ± 2.9	—	—	69.1 ± 2.1	74.9 ± 1.6
Glucagon (0.02 mg/kg)[d]									
Nonpregnant	20	—	24.0 ± 9.2[e]	31.4 ± 16.4	—	11.6 ± 24.9	—	−12.5 ± 15.5	—
36–40 wk	20	—	23.2 ± 5.2	41.8 ± 8.7	—	35.8 ± 14.8	—	12.7 ± 14.6[f]	—
Arginine (0.25 g/lb in 30 min)									(90 min)
Nonpregnant	28	86.1 ± 1.9[c]	—	—	107.9 ± 3.3	—	—	81.5 ± 3.3	75.2 ± 2.6
1st trimester	9	70.5 ± 2.5[f]	—	—	81.4 ± 7.0[f]	—	—	67.5 ± 5.1[f]	72.3 ± 4.2
2d trimester	7	67.5 ± 3.9[f]	—	—	76.4 ± 5.9[f]	—	—	67.4 ± 4.9[f]	71.1 ± 3.8
3d trimester	5	57.7 ± 6.5[f]	—	—	90.9 ± 12.8	—	—	80.9 ± 9.7	72.0 ± 5.6

[a]References: insulin. Burt (1956); tolbutamide. Spellacy et al. (1965c); glucagon. Burt (1957); arginine. Tyson et al. (1969).
[b]Glucose methodology: insulin. Somogyi-Nelson: tolbutamide. Somogyi-Nelson: glucagon. Somogyi-Nelson: arginine. glucose oxidase.
[c]Mean ± SE.
[d]Change from baseline.
[e]Mean ± SD.
[f]Significantly different from nonpregnant ($P < 0.05$ or more).

TABLE 4-17 Insulin Response to 50 g of Oral Glucose at Various Times in Gestation in 19 Healthy Subjects[a]

Gestational Age	Plasma Immunoreactive Insulin (μU/ml)[b] at:							
	0 min	15 min	30 min	45 min	60 min	75 min	90 min	120 min
Nonpregnant[c]	5.8 ± 4.0[d]	27.7 ± 18.2	38.8 ± 18.0	42.0 ± 18.8	32.7 ± 16.1	23.2 ± 12.8	19.5 ± 10.8	13.4 ± 12.5
10 wk	4.2 ± 2.4	28.3 ± 24.8	41.4 ± 24.9	42.6 ± 25.0	34.8 ± 19.7	31.4 ± 20.3	32.0 ± 40.2	16.9 ± 12.6
20 wk	4.2 ± 1.8	27.6 ± 13.9	40.4 ± 25.2	45.3 ± 21.7	38.7 ± 18.8	34.3 ± 15.0	23.4 ± 14.3	15.8 ± 11.0
30 wk[e]	7.6 ± 2.9	37.1 ± 21.7	55.9 ± 37.9	67.1 ± 39.7	61.4 ± 36.8	52.8 ± 32.4	40.6 ± 19.6	22.7 ± 17.2
38 wk[e]	7.8 ± 3.8	37.7 ± 29.3	57.6 ± 35.7	63.0 ± 26.0	66.4 ± 35.2	56.8 ± 22.8	51.6 ± 24.2	28.2 ± 14.9

[a]From Lind et al. (1973).
[b]Single antibody, charcoal adsorption method.
[c]Nonpregnant subjects were the previously pregnant subjects 10–12 wk postpartum: only one subject was lactating.
[d]Mean ± SD.
[e]Fasting level was significantly greater than nonpregnant ($P < 0.01$). Postglucose values were significantly greater than 10 and 20 wk ($P < 0.01$). Postglucose values were significantly greater than nonpregnant ($P < 0.01$).

TABLE 4-18 Insulin Response to 25 g of Glucose Intravenously in the Three Trimesters[a]

References	Gestational Age	Display	Immunoreactive Insulin (μU/ml)[b] at:								
			0 min	15 min	20 min	30 min	40 min	50 min	60 min	90 min	120 min
Spellacy and Goetz (1963); Spellacy et al. (1965a, 1965b)	13–15 wk	x̄	39.0	121.3		80.7			43.5		34.2
		SE	5.1	19.7		11.7			6.1		3.7
	Postpartum	x̄	35.2	95.5		58.5			42.7		37.0
		SE	4.9	21.5		6.1			5.2		4.2
	25–29 wk	x̄	75.8	171.6		127.7			66.5		49.7
		SE	13.4	24.1		21.5			6.4		5.3
	Postpartum	x̄	49.7	84.2		66.3			87.1		48.2
		SE	3.9	6.5		4.4			3.3		3.1
	36–40 wk	x̄	108.7	333.1		222.0			102.0		61.0
		SE	21.0	42.1		46.8			11.8		5.9
	Postpartum	x̄	61.7	117.5		84.5			65.7		57.0
		SE	5.0	12.1		8.0			8.8		5.5
Bleicher et al. (1964)	30–39 wk	x̄	27.6	136.8	128.4	85.3	64.9	47.9	39.9	26.7	
		SE	2.6	17.7	17.7	10.4	6.7	7.0	6.1	5.2	
	Postpartum	x̄	17.1	86.3	71.9	52.7	51.7	34.3	30.1	14.7	
		SE	2.8	12.1	14.6	7.7	9.2	6.4	5.1	4.8	

[a] In the Spellacy and Goetz (1963) and the Spellacy et al. (1965a, 1965b) studies, 20 paired studies were done in each trimester. In the Bleicher et al. (1964) study, 10 paired studies pre- and postpartum were performed. In all of these studies, plasma glucoses were slightly lower in gestation at all time points.
[b] In some of these earlier insulin assays, basal levels tend to run higher than with more current methods (see Tables 4-17 and 4-20).

TABLE 4-19 Special Studies: Insulin Responses to Tolbutamide and Arginine[a]

Study	No.	Immunoreactive Insulin (μU/ml)					
		0 min	15 min	30 min	60 min	90 min	120 min
Tolbutamide (1 g/kg)							
Nonpregnant[b]	12	41 ± 9[c]	85 ± 17	80 ± 15	45 ± 9	—	45 ± 12
36–40 wk	12	59 ± 10	265 ± 56[d]	134 ± 22[d]	81 ± 14[d]	—	87 ± 19[d]
Arginine (0.25 g/lb in 30 min)							
Nonpregnant[e]	28	17.4 ± 1.4	—	90.4 ± 8.6	38.2 ± 6.9	19.0 ± 2.0	—
1st Trimester	9	5.0 ± 2.0[d]	—	20.3 ± 7.4[d]	7.4 ± 3.4[d]	7.2 ± 3.1[d]	—
2nd Trimester	7	7.7 ± 4.4[d]	—	15.4 ± 6.5[d]	7.7 ± 3.6[d]	7.5 ± 4.4[d]	—
3rd Trimester	5	14.8 ± 3.2	—	59.2 ± 15.3	52.6 ± 19.8	24.0 ± 5.2	—

[a]**References**: tolbutamide, Spellacy et al. (1965c); arginine, Tyson et al. (1969).
[b]Paired studies > 6 wk postpartum.
[c]Mean ± SE.
[d]Significantly different from nonpregnant at $P < 0.05$ or greater.
[e]A separate control group not necessarily matched with pregnancy but which is said to be nonobese.

55

TABLE 4-20 Immunoreactive Glucagon (IRG) in Pregnancy and Its Interrelations with Glucose and Immunoreactive Insulin (IRI)[a]

Study	Trimester		4-8 wk Postpartum	Nonpregnant
	2	3		
Fasting levels				
Freinkel et al. (1975)		(25)	(16)	(26)
Glucose (mg/dl)	—	80.0 ± 1.5[b]	87.0 ± 1.4[c]	88.0 ± 0.8[d]
IRI (μU/ml)	—	13.0 ± 1.0	8.2 ± 0.6[d]	6.0 ± 0.3[d]
IRG (pg/ml)	—	60.0 ± 3.0	43.0 ± 3.3[d]	64.0 ± 5.8[e]
Kühl and Holst (1976)	(8)	(8)	(8)	
Glucose (mg/dl)	84.6 ± 1.8	82.6 ± 1.8	84.6 ± 3.6	—
IRI (μU/ml)	6.4 ± 0.6	9.4 ± 1.4[a]	5.0 ± 0.5	—
IRG (pg/ml)	97.5 ± 4.5[c]	153.7 ± 17.2[c]	118.1 ± 10.1	—
IRI/IRG (molar ratio)	1.7 ± 0.2[d]	1.8 ± 0.4[c]	1.1 ± 0.2	—
Postglucose response				
Daniel et al. (1974)		(16)	(16)	
Glucose area (mg min/ml)	—	102.0 ± 6.1	75.0 ± 0.9	—
IRI area (μU min/ml)	—	15,800 ± 1,850	10,900 ± 1,230	—
IRG maximum suppression (%)	—	29.6	15.3	—
Kühl and Holst (1976)	(8)	(8)	(8)	
IRI area (μU min/ml)	3,801 ± 743	5,894 ± 1,502	2,133 ± 343	—
IRG maximum suppression (%)	25.5	24.4	20.0	—

[a]Data of Freinkel et al. (1975), Daniel et al. (1974), and Kühl and Holst (1976). Values in parentheses indicate number of subjects.
[b]Mean ± SEM.
[c]Significant difference second or third trimester versus postpartum, P < 0.05.
[d]Significant difference second or third trimester versus postpartum or nonpregnant, P < 0.01.
[e]Significant difference postpartum versus nonpregnant, P < 0.01.

However, low first and second trimester fasting insulin levels were not seen by all workers (Spellacy and Goetz, 1963; Spellacy *et al.*, 1965a; Edstrom *et al.*, 1974; Kühl and Holst, 1976) and the matter requires further study.

Oral Glucose Tolerance Test

The oral glucose tolerance test has been used many times as a stimulus to insulin secretion in pregnancy. Unfortunately, the data have been presented illustratively rather than as absolute values. However, data for the area under the insulin curve following glucose administration have been recorded. Three examples are given in Table 4-21 and show that a 50–90 percent greater insulin response is seen in third trimester regardless of the glucose dose (Beck and Wells, 1969; Lind *et al.*, 1973; Daniel *et al.*, 1974). Lind *et al.* (1973) have measured insulin levels after the 50-g oral test (Table 4-17). A trend toward elevated insulin levels postglucose is seen late in the test at 10 and 20 wk but is not significant until 30 and 36 wk, coincident with the appearance of clinical insulin resistance (Pedersen, 1967) and the rapid rise in human placental lactogen (HPL) (Samaan *et al.*, 1966).

Intravenous Glucose Tolerance Test

Spellacy and Goetz (1963) and Spellacy *et al.* (1965a, 1965b) have measured insulin secretion in the three trimesters in response to IV glucose: in the first trimester the maximum insulin response is about 40 percent elevated, in the second trimester 2.2-fold, and in the third about 3-fold (Table 4-18). The data of Bleicher *et al.* (1964) (Table 4-18) are shown for comparison inasmuch as the basal insulin level is lower and more representative and blood is drawn at more frequent intervals. In these data, the maximum plasma insulin response is 60 percent greater than the postpartum controls.

Insulin Response to Tolbutamide and Arginine

As shown in Table 4-19, intravenous administration of 1 g of tolbutamide elicits a threefold greater rise in insulin in the third trimester as compared to the nonpregnant control (Spellacy *et al.*, 1965c). By contrast, a hyporesponsiveness of insulin secretion to intravenously administered arginine is seen in the first and second trimesters in the work of Tyson *et al.* (1969). This hyporesponsiveness was confirmed

TABLE 4-21 Integrated Insulin Responses to Oral Glucose Administration in Third-Trimester Pregnant Subjects

References	Glucose Dose (g)	Duration Test (min)	No.	Immunoreactive Insulin (μU min/ml)		
				3rd Trimester[a]	Nonpregnant[b]	P
Beck and Wells (1969)	100	240	14	9,859	5,069	<0.005
Daniel et al. (1974)	100	180	16	15,800 ± 1,850[c]	10,900 ± 1,230	<0.01
Lind et al. (1973)	50	120	19	5,860 ± 675[d]	3,150 ± 1,290	

[a]Antepartum studies were done in the third trimester (Beck and Wells, 1969): 30–40 wk gestation (Daniel et al., 1974); and 38 wk gestation (Lind et al., 1973).
[b]Postpartum subjects were studied after 5 wk (Beck and Wells, 1969): 5–8 wk (Daniel et al., 1974); and 10–12 wk (Lind et al., 1973).
[c]Mean ± SE.
[d]The data of Lind et al. (1973) have been multiplied by 15. Mean ± SD (significance not given).

by King *et al.* (1971) and could be attributed in part to the lower levels of plasma arginine achieved during the infusion. However, King *et al.* (1971) also showed that the plasma insulin response was inappropriately low for the level of plasma arginine achieved in the second trimester. Third-trimester insulin levels were normal (Tyson *et al.*, 1969) or low (King *et al.*, 1971) but not high due again to a low arginine level (King *et al.*, 1971). However, the insulin response was appropriate to the level of arginine achieved compared to nonpregnant controls (King *et al.*, 1971). A similar set of responses in the three trimesters is seen following protein ingestion (Tyson and Merimee, 1970). The mechanisms of these responses and their relationship to the fasting hypoinsulinism of early and midgestation deserve further study.

GLUCAGON SECRETION

Table 4-20 shows the fasting immunoreactive glucagon (IRG) measurements obtained in late human pregnancy with concurrent measures of insulin and glucose (Daniel *et al.*, 1974; Freinkel *et al.*, 1975; Kühl and Holst, 1976). Changes in glucose and insulin are in good agreement in the two studies. The absolute levels of glucagon differ, but this probably reflects differences in immunoassay specificity and technique. Whether or not glucagon is judged to be elevated in late gestation depends upon the basis for comparison. In both studies, glucagon level is elevated in the third trimester relative to postpartum controls. In addition, IRG is higher in third trimester than second trimester in the one study where it was evaluated. However, in the study of Freinkel *et al.* (1975), comparison of third-trimester IRG with a nonpregnant group shows no difference. It may be that IRG is lower in postpartum rather than higher in third trimester and that postpartum comparisons around 6 wk may be premature in certain parameters, as maternal metabolism may not yet be entirely back to normal.

After the administration of glucose, a greater suppression of IRG occurred in gestation in both studies (Daniel *et al.*, 1974; Kühl and Holst, 1976). All of the observations point to a heightened insulin to glucagon ratio in late gestation in both the basal and stimulated state, as has been reported in the laboratory rat (Saudek *et al.*, 1975) and emphasize the anabolic nature of glucoregulation in pregnancy (Saudek *et al.*, 1975). Similar conclusions have been reached by Luyckx *et al.* (1975). An increased insulin to glucagon ratio could contribute to the lower fasting glucose in early gestation, at a time when total demands for glucose are small.

GROWTH HORMONE (HGH)

It took some time before accurate methods to measure growth hormone in pregnancy were developed, because of the cross-reaction of antigrowth hormone antibody with human placental lactogen (Josimovich and MacLaren, 1962). This cross-reaction formed the basis of the earlier discovery of human placental lactogen (Josimovich and MacLaren, 1962). Both of the studies presented in Table 4-22 indicate slight increases in basal HGH as gestation proceeds (Tyson et al., 1969; Yen et al., 1970). This effect probably represents some small HPL contamination, especially since Varma et al. (1971) were able to completely dilute out this effect (see footnote, Table 4-22). Following intravenous arginine or insulin administration, HGH response was reduced in late gestation. Since a reduced HGH release could in part be due to a lesser degree of hypoglycemia or a lesser rise of arginine in the third trimester (King et al., 1971), it is still uncertain if a physiological reduction in HGH secretion in pregnancy really exists.

FREE FATTY ACIDS AND GLYCEROL

A recent study by McDonald-Gibson et al. (1975) indicates a small elevation in FFA in the third trimester relative to the second or first trimesters (Table 4-23), a pattern that has also been observed in the rat (Knopp et al., 1973b). Burt (1960b) found a similar pattern in his initial report on the subject. What is new in the data of McDonald-Gibson et al. (1975) is the very minimal third-trimester rise and the failure of the FFA to fall by 6 wk postpartum. Freinkel et al. (1975) also found only a small third-trimester rise, and Persson and Lunell (1975) report no increase. Why earlier investigators found more prominently elevated levels of FFA throughout gestation remains to be explained. One possible source of artifact is the endogenous hypertriglyceridemia of pregnancy (see below), which, if any test-tube lipolysis were to occur, would cause a higher FFA level in the pregnancy sample. For instance, if plasma samples are not frozen soon after collection but are kept in a refrigerator overnight, the plasma FFA level may double (R. H. Knopp, unpublished observations). Glycerol levels run about one-tenth of the FFA values on a molar basis but show the same trends, lending support to the patterns in plasma FFA reported by McDonald-Gibson et al. (1975). Since increased adipose tissue fatty acid mobilization has been well documented in late gestation in both the rat and man (Knopp et al., 1970; Elliott, 1975), the possibility of an increased fractional turnover of FFA is raised by these observations.

TABLE 4-22 Growth Hormone (HGH) Secretion in Gestation after Intravenous Insulin or Arginine

Study	No.	HGH (ng/ml)[a]					
		0 min	30 min	60 min	90 min	120 min	Maximum Change
Insulin hypoglycemia[b]							
Nonpregnant (0.1 μ/kg)	10	2.5 ± 1.4[d]	4.0 ± 1.3	28.0 ± 5.7	22.5 ± 3.8	15.5 ± 2.8	25.5 ± 5.2
1st Trimester (0.1 μ/kg)	10	4.8 ± 1.2	5.7 ± 1.5	16.2 ± 3.2	17.5 ± 2.9	8.2 ± 1.7	12.7 ± 2.5
2nd Trimester (0.125 μ/kg)	10	6.3 ± 0.9	7.0 ± 0.7	13.5 ± 2.6[e]	10.5 ± 2.1[e]	6.2 ± 2.6[e]	7.2 ± 2.1[e]
3rd Trimester (0.15 μ/kg)	10	5.5 ± 1.0	6.8 ± 1.2	10.5 ± 2.4[e]	7.3 ± 1.4[e]	5.5 ± 1.9[e]	5.0 ± 1.9[e]
Arginine infusion[c]							
Nonpregnant	28	3.4 ± 0.7[d]	18.7 ± 3.6	27.8 ± 3.5	23.7 ± 3.4	—	—
1st Trimester	9	9.8 ± 1.4[e]	37.6 ± 7.1[e]	30.2 ± 4.5	17.4 ± 2.7	—	—
2nd Trimester	7	12.7 ± 1.7[e]	32.4 ± 6.5[e]	40.2 ± 10.2	21.5 ± 3.3	—	—
3rd Trimester	5	12.5 ± 1.0	14.8 ± 2.6	15.8 ± 1.7[e]	15.7 ± 2.3[e]		

[a]Immunoassays for HGH had some cross-reaction with placental lactogen, since HGH values do not rise when antibody reaction with HPL is diluted out [(weeks gestation) mean ± SD in mg/ml]: (6–10) 3.36 ± 1.68, (11–15) 4.95 ± 1.94, (16–20) 4.58 ± 1.75, (21–25) 4.36 ± 1.55, (26–30) 5.65 ± 2.60, (31–35) 4.29 ± 1.46, (36–40) 3.94 ± 1.98, (5–26 subjects). Data of Varma et al. (1971).

[b]Study of Yen et al. (1970). Although insulin doses were increased in succeeding trimesters, 30-min glucose nadirs also increased (mg/100 ml): nonpregnant, 32.4: first trimester, 29.5: 2nd trimester, 35.5; third trimester, 40.5 (Yen et al., 1970).

[c]Study of Tyson et al. (1969).

[d]Mean ± SE.

[e]Significantly different from nonpregnant (P < 0.05 or greater).

61

TABLE 4-23   Plasma Free Fatty Acids (FFA) and Glycerol in Pregnancy[a]

	No.	FFA (μmol/l)	Glycerol (μmol/l)
Nonpregnant[b]	27	428 ± 119[c]	50 ± 17
13 wk	14	413 ± 84	44 ± 14
20 wk	15	370 ± 147	38 ± 9
30 wk	15	336 ± 87	39 ± 14
38 wk	15	422 ± 89[d]	50 ± 18[d]
Postpartum–6 wk	15	468 ± 122	54 ± 17
Postpartum–12 wk	14	383 ± 96	49 ± 14
Postpartum–24 wk	13	328 ± 107	42 ± 12

[a] Data of McDonald-Gibson *et al.* (1975).
[b] Results are for 13–15 women studied serially with a separate nonpregnant control group.
[c] Mean ± SD.
[d] Aggregate values (see McDonald-Gibson *et al.*, 1975) show a significant increase at 38 wk over 30 wk.

KETONE BODIES IN PREGNANCY

Whether or not ketone bodies are elevated after an overnight fast in pregnancy is controversial. The data of Felig and Lynch (1970) indicate a three- to fourfold rise in ketones after overnight fast in the second trimester as compared to controls (Table 4-24). Similar results were reported by Lunell *et al.* (1973) (see footnote, Table 4-24) in nonpregnant young women. In contrast, extensive third-trimester measurements of ketone bodies by Persson and Lunell (1975) in healthy

TABLE 4-24   Ketone Bodies in Pregnancy after Overnight Fast

	Ketone Bodies (mmol/l)			
		Trimester		Start of Labor
Study	Nonpregnant (6)[a]	2 (12)[a]	3 (14)[b]	(8)[c]
Total ketones	–	–	–	0.169 ± 0.040
Acetoacetate	0.06 ± 0.01[d]	0.15 ± 0.03[e]	0.05 ± 0.05	–
β-Hydroxybutyrate	0.10 ± 0.05	0.37 ± 0.04[e]	0.09 ± 0.02	–

[a] Data of Felig and Lynch (1970); enzymatic method.
[b] Data taken from an illustration of Persson and Lunell (1975) at 38 wk gestation, enzymatic method. With respect to B-OHB, not different from 39 nonpregnant women: 0.079 ± 0.011 (Lunell *et al.*, 1973).
[c] Data of Sabata *et al.* (1968).
[d] Mean ± SEM.
[e] Significantly increased over nonpregnant ($P < 0.01$).

mothers discloses no rise compared to the nonpregnant subjects of Felig and Lynch (1970) or Lunell *et al.* (1973). The acetoacetate and β-hydroxybutyrate totals of Persson and Lunell (1975) in the third trimester interestingly correspond closely to the total ketones measured by Sabata *et al.* (1968) at the onset of delivery. In view of the minimal FFA rise in late gestation, a minimal ketone body rise may be occurring but be very hard to measure. There is no question that a striking ketonemia occurs on prolonged fasting in both human and animal pregnancy (Herrera *et al.*, 1969; Felig and Lynch, 1970). What may be at issue are variations in the length of the "overnight" fast. Alternatively, the data may represent genuine differences between second and third trimester. Further studies are required to assess these possibilities.

LIPIDS AND LIPOPROTEINS

Methodology

Since all lipids in the blood plasma are bound to proteins, certain factors affect all lipids in common (see Table 4-25). For instance, upright posture tends to cause hemoconcentration and supine posture tends to lead to hemodilution (Tan *et al.*, 1973; Statland *et al.*, 1974). Likewise, tourniquit stasis is a factor (Statland *et al.*, 1974). The use of an anticoagulant such as EDTA tends to draw water out of red cells, thus diluting the sample as compared to serum. Whether or not the subject has eaten or is fasting at the time the blood is drawn is also an obvious consideration.

With respect to lipid extraction from plasma, a variety of organic solvent systems have been used (Table 4-25). Isopropanol or 2:1 (vol/vol) chloroform methanol are probably the most commonly used at present. These extractions separate the lipids from plasma proteins and other constituents and allow for analysis of the following: total lipids by gravimetry (Wybenga and Inkpen, 1974), phospholipids usually by the molybdenum blue reaction (Wybenga and Inkpen, 1974), triglycerides by measuring the glycerol after saponification (Litchfield, 1972), and cholesterol, usually by the Lieberman-Burchard reaction or the ferric chloride method (Tonks, 1967).

Because they are so frequently performed, the analyses for triglycerides and cholesterol are discussed in greater detail in Table 4-25. The reference methods are the Carlson procedure (Carlson, 1959, 1963) for triglycerides and the Abell-Kendall method (Abell *et al.*, 1952) for cholesterol. Triglyceride measurements vary from lab to lab, often

TABLE 4-25   Guide to Interpreting Triglyceride and Cholesterol
Measurements

---

1. *Effect of posture*

Posture affects blood lipid measurements as well as all proteins and protein-bound
materials in blood. Standing tends to hemoconcentrate and recumbency tends to hemo-
dilute. In one study, recumbency compared to upright posture reduced cholesterol
10.4 percent, and triglyceride, 12.4 percent (Tan *et al.*, 1973). In another study the
same comparison produced an 8.2 percent drop in cholesterol (Statland *et al.*, 1974).
Lesser reductions occur on sitting (2 to 6 percent for cholesterol) (Tan *et al.*, 1973;
Statland *et al.*, 1974). Brief tourniquet application tends to reduce cholesterol 1-2
percent. A longer (3-min) tourniquet application raises cholesterol about 3 percent
(Statland *et al.*, 1974).

2. *Serum versus plasma*

Venous serum or plasma are suitable for lipid determinations. EDTA (1.5 mg/dl of
blood) is the preferred anticoagulant as it has the additional effect of stabilizing
lipoprotein lipids (Lipid Research Clinics Program, 1974). Lipid measurements run
about 3 percent lower in plasma than serum, probably due to the osmotic effect
of EDTA, which draws water out of red cells (personal communication, Russell
Warnick, Clinical Chemist, N.W. Lipid Research Clinic).

3. *Sample preparation*

Lipids are extracted in organic solvents (Litchfield, 1972). Interfering substances including glucose and bilirubin are removed by washing the lipid extract or by adsorption with $CuSO_4$-$Ca(OH)_2$ and Lloyd's reagent. Phospholipids are adsorbed by silicic
acid or zeolite. Mono- and diglycerides are more completely removed by silicic
acid than zeolite. The glyceride extract is then saponified to yield its constituent
glycerol and fatty acids, the glycerol being conveniently measured.

4. *Glyceride glycerol analyses (Litchfield, 1972)*

   a. Manual methods

   (1) Carlson (1959, 1963): This method employs silicic acid adsorption in chloroform methanol and uses chromotropic acid as color reagent. This method or its
automated version is the reference standard.
   (2) Van Handel and Zilversmit (1957): This method employs zeolite adsorption
in chloroform and chromotropic acid for color development (Wybenga and Inkpen,
1974). It tends to run higher than the Carlson method since partial glycerides are
not completely removed. The presence of background color produced by nonsaponi-
fied material in the unknowns may also cause a slightly higher value of a few
percent.

   b. Semiautomated methods

   (1) Autoanalyzer I: The Lofland (1964) method is the semiautomated version
of the chromotropic acid methods.
   (2) Autoanalyzer I: The method of Kessler and Lederer (1965) consists of treat-

TABLE 4-25 (Continued)

ing the isopropanol extract with zeolite, $CuSO_4$-$Ca(OH)_2$, and Lloyd's reagent; saponification; periodate oxidation; and condensation with acetylacetone to produce a fluorescent product. This method may run higher than the Carlson method for reasons discussed under the Van Handel method.

(3) Autoanalyzer II method number 24 of Leon *et al.* (1970): This is an adaptation of the Kessler and Lederer (1965) method.

c. Glycerol kinase enzyme methods

(1) Linked to glycerol phosphate dehydrogenase (Wieland, 1963).

(2) Linked to pyruvate kinase plus lactate dehydrogenase (Wahlefeld *et al.*, 1975). This method corresponds well to AAII in preliminary studies (personal communication with R. Warnick).

5. *Cholesterol analyses (Tonks, 1967)*

a. Manual methods

(1) Bloor: This method was described in 1916; it employs Lieberman-Burchard reagent (acetic anhydride, concentrated sulfuric acid, and glacial acetic acid) in a chloroform lipid extract (Tonks, 1967). Methods by Theorell, Cramer, Lieboff, and King are related (Tonks, 1967).

(2) Abell-Kendall: Abell *et al.* (1952) introduced a saponification step before the Lieberman-Burchard reaction since cholesterol esters produce a greater color intensity than free cholesterol. This is the current reference method (Abell *et al.*, 1952). Methods by Sperry, Keys, and Ham are closely related (Tonks, 1967).

(3) Zlatkis *et al.* (1953) introduced ferric chloride as a color reagent, which reacts to cholesterol and cholesterol ester with equal intensity. There are numerous modifications of this method (Tonks, 1967). Saponification is unnecessary, but the method runs 4–10 percent higher than Abell-Kendall (Tonks, 1967).

(4) Rappaport and Eichorn (1960) used para-toluene sulfonic acid directly on plasma without extraction. This method tends to give higher values than Abell-Kendall and bilirubin interferes.

b. Automated methods

(1) Autoanalyzer I: An automated adaptation of Zak's methods employing isopropanol extract and the ferric chloride-sulfuric acid-acetic acid reagent system (Technicon method N24a) (Block *et al.*, 1966).

(2) Autoanalyzer II: Employs an isopropanol extract and the Lieberman-Burchard reagent (Technicon Autoanalyzer Method File No. 24, 1972). This method is more stable than AAI, but because the saponification step is eliminated the cholesterol esters produce an excessive color reaction. One solution in current use calibrates the AAII against sera standardized in the Abell-Kendall method (Lipid Research Clinics Program, 1974).

(3) Autoanalyzer II, direct method: No extraction is performed; thus, interfering substances in plasma are not removed (Technicon Autoanalyzer Method File No. 24, 1972). Results are 10–15 percent higher than the comparable method by extraction. This is the common method used in clinical laboratories (SMA 6/60 and 12/60 systems) and can lead to an overdiagnosis of hypercholesterolemia.

TABLE 4-25   (Continued)

---

c. Enzyme methods

These are under development and involve production of free cholesterol with a cholesterol esterase, subsequent oxidation by cholesterol oxidase, and coupling with catalase or peroxidase systems to a chromagen as in the glucose oxidase methods (Allain *et al.*, 1974).

---

without obvious explanation. As for cholesterol, the direct method of the SMA 6/60 or 12/60 series may overestimate the cholesterol 10–15 percent for a variety of reasons but mainly because a lipid extract is not made (Table 4-25). Thus, methodology must be considered in the evaluation of results.

Lipid Measurements in Pregnancy

An abundant literature on this subject dates back many years. Table 4-26 reviews the literature from 1934 on, separating the studies into those performed under fasting and nonfasting conditions. The table is constructed to permit comparisons among studies employing varied methods. The consistency of the techniques can be judged from the nonpregnant data. These are surprisingly homogeneous. In the nonfasting group (Table 4-26), total lipids, cholesterol, and phospholipids tend to be higher than those of the fasting group.

In pregnancy, triglycerides increase 2.5- to 4-fold, and cholesterol and phospholipids each increase about 25 percent (Table 4-26). A greater variation is seen in these data than in the nonpregnant group, suggesting that the differences are due to the pregnancies studied rather than the analytical methods. While these data include only third-trimester subjects, important differences can exist within this time interval (see Table 4-27). Racial differences may also be important. The lowest levels of triglyceride and cholesterol and the second lowest phospholipid level in pregnancy are seen in the Nigerian women studied by Taylor (1972). Comparing the racial composition of two American studies, over 90 percent of the subjects of Hillman *et al.* (1975) were Negroes, while those of Montes *et al.* (1976) were almost all Caucasians. Both triglyceride and cholesterol values were higher in the Montes study compared to those of Hillman *et al.* despite the fact that the methodologies were identical and standardized to the same reference methods. This tendency toward higher triglycerides in Caucasians compared to Negroes has been seen in nonpregnant women as well and emphasizes the need for racially specific lipid standards.

Serial Lipid Changes in Pregnancy

Serial changes in plasma lipids over the length of gestation are illustrated in Table 4-27. Two of the three studies suggest a peak at 29–36 wk and then a decline at term. The drop at delivery may be exaggerated in the data of Oliver and Boyd (1955), since earlier measurements were made after subjects had eaten, whereas at delivery subjects were probably postabsorptive. The data of Taylor and Akande (1975) do not show the late downward trend, but the women studied were not very hypercholesterolemic. Phospholipids show a tendency to level off in the third trimester, as do triglycerides, but the data are limited. There is a suggestion of a reduction in cholesterol in the first trimester. Other authors studying individual cases have raised this possibility as well (Peters *et al.*, 1951; Green, 1966). A similar trend is not seen in triglyceride or phospholipid (Table 4-27).

Lipoprotein Lipids

Lipid changes in the major lipoprotein fractions are illustrated in Table 4-28. Prior to 1965, beta lipoproteins referred to the sum of the VLDL and LDL fractions; more recently these have been isolated separately and are termed beta and prebeta (see Knopp *et al.*, 1973a, for review). It can be seen that triglycerides increase two- to fourfold in each of the fractions in pregnancy. The extent of the cholesterol increase in VLDL parallels the triglyceride increase, whereas lesser increases are seen in LDL and HDL cholesterol. In pregnancy, HDL cholesterol measurements are strikingly close in all five studies, and they are higher or unchanged but never lower compared to the nonpregnant. These results contrast with the atherosclerosis-associated hyperlipidemias, where HDL cholesterol is reduced (Fredrickson *et al.*, 1968). Changes in phospholipids mirror those in cholesterol.

Norms for the Lipoprotein Lipids

In order to provide some basis for assessing normal and abnormal for triglyceride and cholesterol in pregnancy, the two SD upper and lower limits for the various fractions have been calculated from data of Montes *et al.* (1976). Of the 30 subjects, all but one were Caucasian. Therefore, the tentative values presented in Table 4-29 are intended for

TABLE 4-26   Plasma Lipids in the Third Trimester of Pregnancy

| | | Plasma Lipids (mg/dl) | | | |
| | | Pregnant | | | |
References	Methods[a]	No.	TL[a]	TG(NF)	TC
Fasting					
Boyd (1934)	TC: Bloor Others: chromic acid oxidation	9	900 ± 130[b]	(353 ± 75)	205 ± 45
Russ et al. (1954)[c]	TC: Bloor PL: F&S	27	–	–	282 ± 62
Konttinen et al. (1964)	TG: Van H TC: Keys (LB) PL: Bartlett	28	–	302 ± 136[b]	345 ± 92
Dannenburg and Burt (1965)	TG: Van H TC: Zak PL: Stewart	17	–	280 ± 22[d]	321[c]
Aurell and Cramér (1966)	TG: Carlson TC: Cramér	18	–	167[g]	258 ± 8
Karsznia and Kaffarnik (1969)	TL: Gravimetric TG: Van H TC: Watson PL: Bartlett	23	1,043 ± 173[b]	284 ± 84	300 ± 70
Fioretti et al. (1970)	TG: Van H TC: Rap PL: Bartlett	23	–	166 ± 18[d]	291 ± 11
Taylor (1972)	TG: Van H TC: Ham PL: King	16	–	120 ± 6[d]	176 ± 5
Knopp et al. (1973a)	TG: K&L TC: AAI	8	–	158 ± 19[d]	200 ± 10
Samsioe et al. (1975)	TG: Carlson TC: Cramér	20	–	180 ± 13[d]	265 ± 8
Hillman et al. (1975)	TG: AAII TG: AAII	38	–	178 ± 74[b]	217 ± 48

PL	EC/TC	Nonpregnant					
		No.	TL	TG(NF)	TC	PL	EC/TC
248 ±43	0.67 ± 0.09	9	617 ± 75	154 ± 77	181 ± 37	195 ± 37	0.70 ± 0.06
372 ± 80	–	21	–	–	189 ± 35	225 ± 28	–
348 ± 57	–	–	–	–	–	–	–
386 ± 13[f]	0.61	17	–	71 ± 5	193[e]	225 ± 13[f]	0.58
283 ± 7	–	18[h]	–	53	162 ± 6	185 ± 4	–
315 ± 59	–	32	645 ± 104	105 ± 22	214 ± 34	226 ± 42	–
565 ± 57	–	12	–	57 ± 2	179 ± 8	170 ± 8	–
224 ± 6	–	23	–	47 ± 7	162 ± 3	185 ± 4	–
–	–	12	–	62 ± 5	160 ± 10	–	–
–	–	18	–	54 ± 4	206 ± 8	–	–
–	–	27[i]	–	86 ± 40	173 ± 34	–	–

TABLE 4-26 (Continued)

		Plasma Lipids (mg/dl)			
		Pregnant			
References	Methods[a]	No.	TL[a]	TG(NF)	TC
Warth *et al.* (1975)	TG: K&L TC: AAI PL: Bartlett	10	–	218 ± 119[b]	213 ± 40
Montes *et al.* (1976)[j]	TG: AAII TC: AAII	30	–	243 ± 15[d]	261 ± 8
Nonfasting Dieckmann and Wegner (1934)	TC: Lieboff	49	–	–	331 ± 9.4[d]
Von Studnitz (1955)	TC: Abell PL: Petersen	10	966 ± 145[b]	–	326 ± 42
Oliver and Boyd (1955)	TC: Sperry	12	–	–	283 ± 60[b]
Watson (1957)	TC: King	39	–	–	243 ± 58[b]
de Alvarez *et al.* (1959)	TL: Gravimetric TC: Sperry PL: F&S	10	1,039 ± 238[b]	–	257 ± 44
Green (1966)	TC: Abell	5	–	–	304
Hashmi and Froze (1972)	TC: Abell	6	–	–	212 ± 14[d]

[a] Abbreviations: *(lipid classes)* TL = total lipid; TG = triglyceride; NF = neutral fat, which is roughly equivalent to TG; TC = total cholesterol; EC = esterified cholesterol; PL = phospholipids; *(methods)* Van H = Van Handel; LB = Lieberman-Burchard; Rap = Rappaport and Eichorn; K&L = Kessler and Lederer, AA = autoanalyzer; F&S = Fiske and Subbarow.

[b] Mean ± SD.

[c] Samples were obtained at delivery and are assumed to be fasting.

[d] Mean ± SE.

		Nonpregnant					
PL	EC/TC	No.	TL	TG(NF)	TC	PL	EC/TC
263 ± 62	–	10	–	54 ± 32	189 ± 40	207 ± 41	–
–	–	30	–	78 ± 6	203 ± 4	–	–
–	–	–	–	–	–	–	–
398 ± 111	–	10	664 ± 124	–	200 ± 33	242 ± 28	–
–	–	12	–	–	201 ± 45	–	–
–	–	38	–	–	228 ± 43	–	–
357 ± 39	–	8	761 ± 232	–	212 ± 44	299 ± 26	–
		5	–	–	198	–	–
217 ± 27	–	–	–	–	–	–	–

ᵉSum of free and esterified cholesterols.
ᶠData originally presented as lipid phosphorus are converted to phospholipid by multiplying by 25.
ᵍData originally presented as mmol/l are converted to mg/dl using the molecular weight of triolein (885.5).
ʰSame subjects studied 9 mo postpartum.
ⁱPostpartum subjects not taking oral contraceptives are most >12 wk postpartum.
ʲUnpublished data of A. Montes and R. H. Knopp. At 6 wk postpartum, no subjects were taking oral contraceptives.

TABLE 4-27 Serial Lipid Measurements in Pregnancy (mg/dl)[a]

References	Diet	NP	Weeks Gestation									Post-partum
			0–8	9–12	13–16	17–20	21–24	25–28	29–32	33–36	37–40	
Total Lipid												
de Alvarez et al. (1959)	Fed	(20)[b] 711 ± 139[c]	(2) 688 ± 105	(4) 653 ± 33	(8) 694 ± 148	(13) 745 ± 105	(10) 737 ± 55	(12) 900 ± 198	(9) 964 ± 208	(10) 1018 ± 194	(8) 1039 ± 239	(20) 711 ± 139
Triglyceride												
Svanborg and Vikrot (1965)	Fast	–	–	33[d]	62	–	113	122	170	244	228	–
	Fed	–	–	64[d]	71	44	95	95	140	166	–	–
Karsznia and Kaffarnik (1969)	Fast	(32) 105 ± 22[c]	–	–	104 ± 33	–	–	147 ± 54	–	–	284 ± 84	
Cholesterol												
Oliver and Boyd (1955)	Fed	–	–	(12) 187 ± 35[c]	(9) 189 ± 42	(10) 207 ± 31	(11) 211 ± 38	(10) 239 ± 56	(12) 282 ± 57	(12) 283 ± 60	(12) 239 ± 56[e]	(12) 201 ± 45
de Alvarez et al. (1959)	Fed	(15) 178 ± 35[c]	(2) 200 ± 51	(4) 152 ± 41					(8) 266 ± 58	(9) 257 ± 44	(4) 249 ± 44	(8) 212 ± 44
Taylor and Akande (1975)	Fast	–		(12) 166 ± 40[f]	(24) 175 ± 26	(16) 207 ± 21	(21) 196 ± 28	(10) 209 ± 21	(5) 209 ± 16	(9) 205 ± 27	(2) 210 ± 16	–
Phospholipid												
de Alvarez et al. (1959)	Fed	(15) 256 ± 36[c]	(2) 240	(4) 263 ± 37	(9) 258 ± 55	(12) 278 ± 64	(11) 282 ± 49	(10) 333 ± 49	(8) 346 ± 48	(9) 357 ± 39	(4) 350 ± 16	(8) 299 ± 26
Taylor and Akande (1975)	Fast	–		(12) 187 ± 41[f]	(24) 203 ± 48	(12) 207 ± 38	(22) 212 ± 33	(15) 206 ± 36	(10) 231 ± 42	(9) 227 ± 33	–	–

[a]Representative studies are presented.
[b]Values in parentheses indicate number of subjects.
[c]Mean ± SD.
[d]Results converted from millimoles to mg/100 ml using molecular weight of triolein = 885.5.
[e]Samples taken at delivery and therefore probably fasting.
[f]The highest of three socioeconomic strata of Nigerian women.

TABLE 4-28 Lipoprotein Lipids after Overnight Fast in the Third Trimester of Pregnancy (mg/dl)[a]

References	Pregnant				Nonpregnant			
	No.	Beta		Alpha (HDL)	No.	Beta		Alpha (HDL)
		VLDL	LDL			VLDL	LDL	
Triglycerides								
Aurell and Cramér (1966)	18	–	127	23	18	–	54	7
Hillman et al. (1975)	38	86 ± 55[b]	52 ± 19	35 ± 8	27	48 ± 35	22 ± 6	9 ± 4
Warth et al. (1975)	10	129 ± 105[b]	59 ± 15	35 ± 17	10	31 ± 19	23 ± 8	12 ± 4
Montes and Knopp[c]	30	121 ± 11[d]	81 ± 6	29 ± 2	30	31 ± 5	28 ± 2	9 ± 1
Cholesterol								
Russ et al. (1954)	27	–	207 ± 59	63 ± 18	21	–	123 ± 32	61 ± 13[e]
Aurell and Cramér (1966)	10	–	185 ± 9[d]	64 ± 4	10	–	118 ± 5	45 ± 2[f]
Hillman et al. (1975)	38	17 ± 15[b]	126 ± 45	62 ± 14	27	13 ± 14	108 ± 31	48 ± 12[g]
Warth et al. (1975)	10	30 ± 17[b]	98 ± 38	61 ± 18	10	9 ± 3	91 ± 21	75 ± 22[e]
Montes and Knopp[c]	30	25 ± 2[d]	171 ± 9	61 ± 3	30	8 ± 1	125 ± 4	61 ± 3[h]
Phospholipid								
Russ et al. (1954)	27	–	206 ± 53[b]	139 ± 34	21	–	98 ± 23	117 ± 20
Aurell and Cramér (1966)	18	–	170 ± 8[d]	117 ± 8	18	–	93 ± 5	98 ± 4
Warth et al. (1975)	10	43 ± 33[b]	85 ± 17	131 ± 30	10	14 ± 7	66 ± 17	138 ± 30

[a]Abbreviations: VLDL, very-low-density lipoprotein; LDL, low-density lipoprotein; HDL, high-density lipoprotein (usually ρ = 1.006–1.063; however, for Cramér this fraction is ρ < 1.063): HDL, high-density lipoprotein (ρ = 1.063–1.21 and also corresponds to alpha lipoprotein). VLDL plus LDL = beta lipoprotein in this older usage.
[b]Mean ± SD.
[c]Previously unpublished data of Montes and Knopp.
[d]Mean ± SE.
[e]Nonpregnant subjects.
[f]Nine months postpartum.
[g]Most subjects tested after 12 wk gestation.
[h]Six weeks postpartum; 20 wk postpartum the HDL cholesterol in these subjects was 54 ± 2 in lactating subjects and 44 ± 6 in nonlactating, non-oral-contraceptive-taking subjects.

TABLE 4-29   Tentative Two SD Upper and Lower Limits for Plasma
Triglyceride and Cholesterol in Third Trimester Pregnancy
(mean, 36 wk) and 6 wk Postpartum[a]

	Pregnant (36 wk)		Postpartum (6 wk)	
Test	Lower Limit[b]	Upper Limit[b]	Lower Limit	Upper Limit
Triglyceride				
Total	131	416	33	166
VLDL[c]	55	231	4	161
LDL[c]	31	150	13	53
HDL[c]	27	60	3	14
Cholesterol				
Total	177	345	157	227
VLDL	0	51	0	18
LDL	78	264	80	170
HDL	32	90	31	91

[a]Previously unpublished data of Montes and Knopp. Studies were done between 30 and 40 wk gestation and 6 wk
postpartum. Twenty-three of the postpartum subjects were lactating, and seven were not. There are no differences
between the two groups postpartum. Twenty-nine were Caucasians, and one was black. In non-oral-contraceptive-
taking subjects, results are identical after 20 wk postpartum except for a drop in HDL cholesterol (see Table 4-28).
Methodology for triglyceride and cholesterol is based on autoanalyzer II techniques. Fractionations were performed
according to methods of the Lipid Research Clinics Program (1974).
[b]All values represent the 2 SD upper or lower limit; 2.5 percent of the population exceeds each limit. These limits
are only tentative and are to be used only as a general guideline until data from larger numbers of subjects are
available and the fifth and ninety-fifth percentiles can be calculated. For triglyceride, the 2 SD limits are based on
$\log_{10}$-transformed data.
[c]VLDL = very-low-density lipoprotein; LDL = low-density lipoprotein; HDL = high-density lipoprotein.

use primarily in Caucasian subjects and when lipid measurements are
done using AAII methodology. These data will be useful until studies
with larger numbers of subjects are available.

Lipoprotein Lipid Composition

When lipoprotein lipid composition is analyzed (Table 4-30), two
distinct patterns are seen (Warth *et al.*, 1975). Increases in all constituents of VLDL and IDL are proportional, maintaining constant the
percentage composition of the lipids in these two fractions. By contrast, LDL$_2$ and HDL show greater increases in triglyceride than the
other lipids, leading to a percentage shift in the direction of triglyceride. The compositional studies suggest that VLDL and IDL are
metabolized as a unit and that there may be some similarities in the
metabolism of LDL$_2$ and HDL as well (Warth *et al.*, 1975).

TABLE 4-30 Effect of Third-Trimester Pregnancy on Plasma Lipoprotein Lipid Percentage Composition[a]

Test	Percentage Composition		
	Pregnant	Control	P
VLDL[b]	(10)[c]	(10)	
Triglyceride	63.0 ± 4.1[d]	53.7 ± 14.5	NS
Cholesterol	15.7 ± 3.7	18.5 ± 5.7	NS
Phospholipid	21.4 ± 2.5	26.5 ± 13.5	NS
IDL ($\rho = 1.006-1.019$)	(5)	(5)	
Triglyceride	35.0 ± 8.4	43.4 ± 18.3	NS
Cholesterol	33.6 ± 7.0	25.8 ± 6.1	NS
Phospholipid	31.8 ± 5.9	30.6 ± 14.2	NS
LDL$_2$ ($\rho = 1.019-1.063$)	(5)	(5)	
Triglyceride	24.2 ± 6.5	11.2 ± 2.9	<0.01
Cholesterol	38.6 ± 9.4	51.0 ± 1.7	<0.05
Phospholipid	37.9 ± 7.5	38.2 ± 2.6	NS
HDL	(10)	(10)	
Triglyceride	15.1 ± 4.4	5.3 ± 2.3	<0.001
Cholesterol	26.7 ± 4.3	33.3 ± 5.8	<0.01
Phospholipid	58.1 ± 3.6	61.8 ± 4.8	NS

[a] Data of Warth et al. (1975).
[b] Abbreviations: VLDL = very-low-density lipoprotein ($\rho < 1.006$), IDL = intermediate-density lipoprotein ($\rho = 1.006-1.019$), LDL$_2$ = low-density lipoprotein$_2$ ($\rho = 1.019-1.063$), HDL = high-density lipoprotein ($\rho > 1.063$).[2]
[c] Number of subjects.
[d] Mean ± SD.

Apolipoproteins

Complete studies of apolipoproteins in pregnancy have been performed by Schonfeld's group and our own and are presented in Table 4-31 (Schonfeld and Pfleger, 1974; Hillman et al., 1975; Montes et al., 1976). With respect to apolipoprotein B the data are in reasonable agreement, showing the greatest increase in VLDL. A less dramatic increase in apolipoprotein AI is seen in the data of Montes et al. (1976) compared to the data of Schonfeld and Pfleger (1974). The data of Montes should be more accurate since a more quantitative delipidation step is used in the Albers method (Albers et al., 1976) for apo AI immunoassay. A decrease in apolipoprotein CII relative to CIII$_2$ was detected by Montes et al. (1976) probably because of the superiority of the Kane (1973) method of delipidation and electrophoresis. As CII is an activator and CIII an inhibitor of lipoprotein lipase, the implication is that lipoprotein lipase regulated removal of VLDL triglycerides should be reduced in late gestation.

TABLE 4-31 Plasma Apolipoproteins after Overnight Fast in Third Trimester of Pregnancy

References	Pregnancy				Nonpregnant			
	No.	VLDL	LDL	HDL	No.	VLDL	LDL	HDL
Apolipoprotein B (mg/100 ml)								
Hillman et al. (1975)	38	7 ± 4[a]	91 ± 25	–	38[b]	3 ± 1	84 ± 60	–
Montes et al. (1976)[c]	30	21 ± 2[d]	95 ± 7	–	30[e]	4 ± 1	116 ± 5	–
Apolipoprotein A_1 (mg/100 ml)								
Schonfeld and Pfleger (1974)	22	–	–	197 ± 36[a]	34	–	–	104 ± 34
Montes et al. (1976)[c]	30	–	–	165 ± 3[d]	30[e]	–	–	123 ± 4
Apolipoprotein C (%)								
Hillman et al. (1975)	4				4			
CII		19 ± 2[a]	–	–		21 ± 3	–	–
$CIII_1$		48 ± 1	–	–		45 ± 4	–	–
$CIII_2$		33 ± 1	–	–		34 ± 5	–	–
Montes et al. (1976)[c]	29				16			
CII		18 ± 1[d]	–	–		28 ± 1[f]	–	–
$CIII_1$		44 ± 1	–	–		43 ± 1	–	–
$CIII_2$		38 ± 1	–	–		28 ± 2[f]	–	–

[a] Mean ± SD.
[b] Postpartum subjects include 11 taking oral contraceptives. Most subjects were studied >12 wk postpartum.
[c] Data of Montes et al. (1976). Differences from Schonfeld and Pfleger (1974) and Hillman et al. (1975) probably are methodological. See text for details.
[d] Mean ± SE.
[e] Postpartum studies all done at 6 wk. At 20 wk postpartum, apoB levels were 99 ± 3 mg/dl in non-oral-contraceptive-taking subjects.
[f] Significantly different from pregnant, $P < 0.001$. These studies represent pooled data from subjects studied 6 or 20 wk postpartum, there being no difference between the two times.

Total Lipoproteins

An assessment of total lipoprotein changes in pregnancy can be appreciated from data obtained using the analytical ultracentrifuge (Table 4-32). The results obtained by Gofman and associates (1954) and generally confirmed in the data of Barclay (1972) are compatible with the results of individual lipoprotein constituents already presented. The greatest increase is in the Sf 20–100 fraction, which corresponds to the increases in the VLDL lipid and apoprotein already described.

Fatty Acid Composition

Analysis of fatty acid composition in pregnancy is of interest in that it provides information on the importance of synthesis of endogenous fat (saturated fatty acids) versus exogenous fat (polyunsaturated fatty acids), assuming removal to be the same. In general, the saturated fatty acids become more abundant relative to the polyunsaturated fatty acids in late gestation as reported by de Alvarez *et al.* (1967) and confirmed in lecithin by Samsioe *et al.* (1975). New information is provided by Taylor (1972), who finds an exaggeration of this trend in midgestation (Table 4-33). These data suggest that the greatest amount of endogenous fat synthesis occurs in midgestation, an idea proposed elsewhere based on data from animal models (Knopp *et al.*, 1975). Partly on this basis, we have speculated that the hyperlipidemia of pregnancy is due to lipid overproduction in midgestation with an additional element of underremoval near term (Knopp *et al.*, 1975).

Carbohydrate Induction Studies

In a further attempt to understand the basis for the hyperlipidemia of pregnancy, we have studied four pregnant subjects in the third trimester before and after high carbohydrate feeding. Ordinarily, an increase in triglycerides is induced that is 50 to 100 percent of the baseline triglyceride (Glueck *et al.*, 1969). In this study by Warth and Knopp (1977), only a 9 percent increase in total triglyceride was detected, which in itself is not significant (Table 4-34). By contrast, postpartum studies in two subjects showed a 63 percent increase in total triglycerides. These data point to a "resistance" to dietary exacerbation of hypertriglyceridemia and suggest a primacy of hormonal mechanisms. Nonetheless, at least two reports suggest a reduction in plasma lipids during pregnancy in poorly nourished individuals (Hashmi and Afroze, 1972; Taylor and Akande, 1975). The possibility that *reduced* maternal lipids may reflect poor maternal nutrition deserves further study.

TABLE 4-32 Total Lipoprotein in Various Fractions as Determined in the Analytical Ultracentrifuge

| | | Total Lipoprotein (mg/dl) | | | | | | |
| | | Sf° | | | | HDL | | |
References	No. of Subjects	100–400[a]	20–100	12–20	0–12	1	2	3
Gofman et al. (1954)[b]								
Pregnant	9	34.2	141.3	105.2	369.2	21.7	151.0	254.7
Nonpregnant	9	20.9	56.4	47.7	298.6	15.1	121.0	207.0
P		NS	<0.05	<0.05	<0.05	<0.05	NS	<0.01
Barclay (1972)[b]								
Pregnant								
(24 wk)		54	122	112	535		102	213
(30 wk)		11	107	131	568		112	250
Nonpregnant		2	3	18	389		133	126
		0	3	6	339		161	126

[a]Flotation ranges approximate the following density fractions: VLDL = Sf° 20–400, LDL = Sf° 0–20, IDL (LDL₁) = Sf° 12–20, LDL₂ = Sf° 0–12, HDL₁ = HDL lipoproteins at $\rho < 1.063$, HDL₂ = ρ of 1.063–1.125, HDL₃ = ρ of 1.125–1.25.
[b]Dietary status was not specified in these studies, and subjects are presumed to be nonfasting.

TABLE 4-33   Serum Fatty Acid Composition in Pregnancy

Test	Fatty Acid Composition (%)		
	NP	Wk 24	Wk 36
Total fatty acids			
(Data of Taylor, 1972)	(23)[a]	(12)	(16)
16:0	28.4 ± 0.7[b]	32.5 ± 0.8	30.0 ± 0.5[c]
16:1	4.0 ± 0.3	3.5 ± 0.4	2.8 ± 0.1
18:0	8.3 ± 0.4	8.3 ± 0.5	6.2 ± 0.1[c]
18:1	26.0 ± 0.7	27.6 ± 0.8	27.0 ± 0.6
18:2	23.6 ± 0.8	19.6 ± 0.9	22.6 ± 0.6[c]
20:0	1.0 ± 0.2	1.5 ± 0.5	0.9 ± 0.3
20:2	0.8 ± 0.3	0.1 ± 0.1	1.4 ± 0.3
20:3	0.1 ± 0.2	0	0.2 ± 0.1
20:4	3.1 ± 0.2	2.9 ± 0.2	3.9 ± 0.2[c]
Saturated fatty acid	38.3 ± 0.9	42.9 ± 1.2	37.8 ± 0.4
Monounsaturated fatty acid	30.0 ± 0.6	31.1 ± 1.1	29.8 ± 0.4
Polyunsaturated fatty acid	26.7 ± 1.5	22.6 ± 1.0	26.7 ± 0.6
Phosphatidyl choline fatty acids			
(Data of Samsioe et al., 1975)	(18)		(20)[d]
16:0	29.6 ± 0.3[b]	–	37.4 ± 0.4
16:1	0.7 ± 0.1	–	1.0 ± 0.0
18:0	13.9 ± 0.2	–	9.5 ± 0.2
18:1	11.7 ± 0.2	–	12.7 ± 0.3
18:2	28.5 ± 0.7[e]	–	24.9 ± 0.4[e]
20:3	2.1 ± 0.2	–	2.8 ± 0.1
20:4	6.7 ± 0.3	–	5.7 ± 0.3
22:6	4.2 ± 0.3	–	4.0 ± 0.2

[a] Values in parenthesis indicate number of subjects.
[b] Mean ± SE.
[c] Wk 24 and 36 are significantly different ($P < 0.01$).
[d] Mean gestational age = 33.6 wk.
[e] 18:2 is relatively decreased in gestation but in absolute terms is significantly increased (mg/100 ml): (NP) 57.1 versus (R) 65.2 ($P < 0.01$).

TABLE 4-34   Effect of Pregnancy on Triglyceride
Response to High Carbohydrate Feeding[a]

	Triglyceride Increase[b]			
	mg/dl		%	
Test	3d Trimester	6 wk Postpartum[c]	3d Trimester	6 wk Postpartum[c]
	(4)[d]	(2)	(4)	(2)
Total plasma	13 ± 16^e	48 ± 18	9 ± 10	41 ± 10^f
VLDL	14 ± 6	53 ± 19^f	17 ± 6	68 ± 19^g
HDL	3 ± 2	4 ± 1	11 ± 9	21 ± 6

[a] Data of Warth and Knopp (1977). Dietary regimen consisted of 3 days of standard diet (40% carbohydrate, 45% fat, 15% protein) followed by 5–7 days of high carbohydrate diet (75% carbohydrate, 5% fat, 15% protein).
[b] Increase is calculated as the difference between the last two days of baseline diet compared to days 4–7 of the test diet.
[c] The subjects studied postpartum are among the four studied antepartum.
[d] Values in parentheses indicate number of subjects.
[e] Mean ± SE.
[f] Postpartum result greater than antepartum., $P < 0.06$. In the two paired studies, postpartum increases were consistently greater than antepartum.
[g] Postpartum result greater than antepartum, $P < 0.025$.

SUMMARY

Table 4-35 presents norms for metabolic parameters in pregnancy that are reasonably well documented. These include standards for fasting and postprandial glucose, the 1-h 50-g glucose screening test, the oral and intravenous glucose tolerance tests, and fasting plasma triglycerides and cholesterol. Still lacking are norms for ketone bodies and polypeptide hormones in pregnancy. These needs and the general goal that all babies born be healthy as population growth declines should spur further research on nutrition and metabolism in pregnancy.

ACKNOWLEDGMENTS

Portions of this study were supported by contract #NO1-VN12157 from the Lipid Research Clinics Program, grant HD-08968-02, and the National Academy of Sciences. We are grateful to Drs. Paul Beck, Ronald Kalkhoff, John B. O'Sullivan, and William N. Spellacy for their reviews of the manuscript and the typing assistance of Ms. Linda Lillard.

TABLE 4-35 Summary of Diagnostic Norms for Metabolic Studies in Pregnancy[a]

Test	Whole Blood (mg/dl)		Plasma (mg/dl)	
	Lower Limit	Upper Limit	Lower Limit	Upper Limit
Glucose				
Fasting	—	90	—	103
Postprandial (morning)				
0.5–1 h	—	114	—	130
1–2 h	—	105	—	120
2–3 h	—	94	—	107
3–4 h	—	92	—	105
>4 h	—	84	—	96
Screening (50 g of glucose, draw blood 1 h later)	—	130	—	148
Oral GTT (100 g) (any 2 values constitute an abnormal test)				
0 h	—	90	—	103
1 h	—	165	—	188
2 h	—	145	—	165
3 h	—	125	—	143
Intravenous GTT (25 g) (k value)	1.13	—	1.13	—
Lipids (tentative)[b]				
Triglyceride (total)	—	—	131	416
Cholesterol (total)	—	—	177	345

[a]All values represent the 2 SD upper or lower limit for subjects in the second and third (oral GTT) or third trimesters (all of the other tests).
[b]The lipid values are for tentative use (primarily in Caucasians) until data from larger studies are available.

REFERENCES

Abell, L. L., B. B. Levy, B. B. Brodie, and F. E. Kendall. 1952. A simplified method for estimation of total cholesterol in serum and demonstration of its specificity. J. Biol. Chem. 195:357–366.

ADA Committee on Statistics. 1969. Standardization of the oral glucose tolerance test. Diabetes 18:299–307.

Albers, J. J., F. W. Wahl, V. G. Cabana, W. R. Hazzard, and J. J. Hoover. 1976. Quantitation of apoprotein Al of human plasma high density lipoprotein. Metabolism 25:633–644.

Allain, C. C., L. S. Poon, C. S. G. Chan, W. Richmond, and P. C. Fu. 1974. Enzymatic determination of total serum cholesterol. Clin. Chem. 20:470–475.

Amatuzio, D. S., F. L. Stutzman, M. J. Vanderbilt, and S. Nesbitt. 1953. Interpretation of the rapid intravenous glucose tolerance test in normal individuals and in mild diabetes mellitus. J. Clin. Invest. 32:428–435.

Aurell, M., and K. Cramér. 1966. Serum lipids and lipoproteins in human pregnancy. Clin. Chim. Acta 13:278–284.

Barclay, M. 1972. Lipoprotein class distribution in normal and diseased states. pp. 585–704. *In* G. J. Nelson, ed., Blood Lipids and Lipoproteins. Wiley-Interscience, New York.

Beck, P., and S. A. Wells. 1969. Comparison of the mechanisms underlying carbohydrate intolerance in subclinical diabetic women during pregnancy and during postpartum oral contraceptive steroid treatment. J. Clin. Endocrinol. Metab. 29:807–818.

Billewicz, W. Z., J. Anderson, and T. Lind. 1973. New index for evaluation of oral glucose tolerance test results. Br. Med. J. 1:573–577.

Billis, A., and G. K. Rastogi. 1966. Studies in methods of investigating carbohydrate. Diabetologia 2:169–177.

Bleicher, S. J., J. B. O'Sullivan, and N. Freinkel. 1964. Carbohydrate metabolism in pregnancy. V. The interrelations of glucose, insulin and free fatty acids in late pregnancy and postpartum. N. Engl. J. Med. 271:866–872.

Block, W. D., K. J. Jarrett, and J. B. Levine. 1966. An automated determination of serum total cholesterol with a single color reagent. Clin. Chem. 12:681–689.

Boyd, E. M. 1934. The lipemia of pregnancy. J. Clin. Invest. 13:347–363.

Brunzell, J. D., R. L. Lerner, W. R. Hazzard, D. Porte, and E. L. Bierman. 1971. Improved glucose tolerance with high carbohydrate feeding in mild diabetes. N. Engl. J. Med. 284:521–524.

Burt, R. L. 1956. Peripheral utilization of glucose in pregnancy. III. Insulin tolerance. Obstet. Gynecol. 7:658–664.

Burt, R. L. 1957. Carbohydrate metabolism in pregnancy. Observations on glucagon (hyperglycemic-glycogenolytic factor) in normal pregnancy and the puerperium. Am. J. Obstet. Gynecol. 74:551–558.

Burt, R. L. 1958. Reactivity to tolbutamide in normal pregnancy. Obstet. Gynecol. 12:447–453.

Burt, R. L. 1960a. Carbohydrate metabolism in pregnancy. Clin. Obstet. Gynecol. 3:310–325.

Burt, R. L. 1960b. Plasma nonesterified fatty acids in normal pregnancy and the puerperium. Obstet. Gynecol. 15:460–464.

Carey, R. N., D. Feldbrueggue, and J. D. Westgard. 1974. Evaluation of the adaptation of the glucose oxidase/peroxidase-3-methyl-2-benzothiazolinone hydrazine-N,

N-dimethylalanine procedure to the Technician "SMA 12/60" and comparison with other automated methods for glucose. Clin. Chem. 20:595–602.

Carlson, L. 1959. Determination of serum glycerides. Acta Soc. Med. Ups. 64:208–213.

Carlson, L. 1963. Determination of serum triglycerides. J. Atheroscler. Res. 3:334–336.

Cornblath, M., and R. Schwartz. 1966. Disorders of carbohydrate metabolism in infancy. W. B. Saunders, Co., Philadelphia. 297 pp.

Daniel, R. R., B. E. Metzger, N. Freinkel, G. R. Faloona, R. H. Unger, and M. Nitzan. 1974. Carbohydrate metabolism in pregnancy. XI. Response of plasma glucagon to overnight fast and oral glucose during normal pregnancy and in gestational diabetes. Diabetes 23:771–776.

Dannenburg, W. N., and R. L. Burt. 1965. The effect of insulin and glucose on plasma lipids during pregnancy and the puerperium. Am. J. Obstet. Gynecol. 92:195–201.

Davison, J. M., and F. E. Hytten. 1975. Renal handling of glucose in pregnancy, pp. 2–18. *In* H. W. Sutherland and J. M. Stowers, eds., Carbohydrate Metabolism in Pregnancy and The Newborn. Churchill Livingstone, New York.

Davison, J. M., and C. Lovedale. 1974. The excretion of glucose during normal pregnancy and after delivery. J. Obstet. Gynaecol. Br. Commonw. 51:30–34.

de Alvarez, R. R., D. F. Gaiser, D. M. Simkins, E. K. Smith, and G. E. Bratvold. 1959. Serial studies of serum lipids in normal human pregnancy. Am. J. Obstet. Gynecol. 77:743–759.

de Alvarez, R. R., B. W. Goodell, and I. Zighelboim. 1967. Fatty acid composition of serum lipids in pregnancy and gynecologic cancer. Am. J. Obstet. Gynecol. 97:419–442.

Dieckmann, W. J., and C. R. Wegner. 1934. Studies of the blood in normal pregnancy. VI. Plasma cholesterol in milligrams per hundred cubic centimeters, gram per kilogram and variations in total amount. Arch. Intern. Med. 53:540–550.

Edstrom, K., E. Cerasi, and R. Luft. 1974. Insulin response to glucose infusion during pregnancy. A prospective study of high and low insulin responders with normal carbohydrate tolerance. Acta Endocrinol. 75:87–104.

Elliott, J. A. 1975. The effect of pregnancy on the control of lipolysis in fat cells isolated from human adipose tissue. Eur. J. Clin. Invest. 5:159–164.

Felig, P., and V. Lynch. 1970. Starvation in human pregnancy: hypoglycemia, hypoinsulinemia, and hyperketonemia. Science 170:990–992.

Fioretti, P., A. R. Genazzani, M. L. Aubert, G. Gragnoli, and A. Pupillo. 1970. Correlation between human chorionic somatomammotropin (lactogen), immunoreactive insulin, glucose, and lipid fractions in plasma of pregnant women. J. Obstet. Gynaecol. Br. Commonw. 77:745–751.

Fredrickson, D. S., R. I. Levy, and F. T. Lindgren. 1968. A comparison of heritable abnormal lipoprotein patterns as defined by two different techniques. J. Clin. Invest. 47:2446–2457.

Freinkel, N. 1965. Effects of the conceptus on maternal metabolism during pregnancy, pp. 679–691. *In* G. S. Liebel and C. A. Wrenshall, eds., On the Nature and Treatment of Diabetes. Excerpta Medica Foundation, Amsterdam.

Freinkel, N., B. E. Metzger, M. Nitzan, R. Daniel, B. Z. Surmaczynska, and T. C. Nagel. 1975. Facilitated anabolism in late pregnancy: some novel maternal compensations for accelerated starvation, pp. 474–488. *In* W. J. Malaisse and J. Pirart, eds., Proceedings of the Eighth Congress of the International Diabetes Federation. Excerpta Medica, Amsterdam.

Gillmer, M. D. G., R. W. Beard, F. M. Brooke, and N. W. Oakley. 1975. Carbohydrate metabolism in pregnancy. I. Diurnal plasma glucose profile in normal and diabetic women. Br. Med. J. iii:399–402.

Glueck, C. J., R. I. Levy, and D. S. Fredrickson. 1969. Immunoreactive insulin, glucose tolerance and carbohydrate inducibility in type II, III, IV, and V hyperlipidemia. Diabetes 18:739–747.

Gochman, N., and J. M. Schmitz. 1972. Application of a new peroxide indicator reaction to the specific, automated determination of glucose with glucose oxidase. Clin. Chem. 18:943–950.

Gofman, J. W., O. DeLalla, F. Glazier, N. K. Freeman, F. T. Lindgren, A. V. Nichols, B. Strisower, and A. R. Tamplin. 1954. The serum lipoprotein transport system in health, metabolic disorders, atherosclerosis and coronary heart disease. Plasma 2:413–484.

Green, J. G. 1966. Serum cholesterol changes in pregnancy. Am. J. Obstet. Gynecol. 95:387–393.

Guttorm, E. 1974. Practical screening for diabetes mellitus in pregnant women. Acta Endocrinol. Suppl. 182:11–24.

Hashmi, J. A., and N. Afroze. 1972. Plasma fibrinogen and serum lipids in anemia of pregnancy. Am. J. Obstet. Gynecol. 112:821–826.

Herrera, E., R. H. Knopp, and N. Freinkel. 1969. Carbohydrate metabolism in pregnancy. VI. Plasma fuels, insulin, liver composition, gluconeogenesis, and nitrogen metabolism during late gestation in the fed and fasted rat. J. Clin. Invest. 48:2260–2272.

Hillman, L., G. Schonfeld, J. P. Miller, and G. Wulff. 1975. Apolipoproteins in human pregnancy. Metabolism 24:943–952.

Hytten, F. E., and I. Leitch. 1971. The Physiology of Human Pregnancy, 2nd ed. Blackwell Scientific Publications, Oxford. 599 pp.

Hytten, F. E., and T. Lind. 1973. Diagnostic Indices in Pregnancy. Ciba-Geigy Ltd., Basel. 122 pp.

Jackson, W. P. U. 1965. Effects of pregnancy on glucose tolerance, pp. 718–721. *In* B. S. Liebel and G. A. Wrenshall, eds., On the Nature and Treatment of Diabetes. Excerpta Medica Foundation, Amsterdam.

Josimovich, J. B., and J. A. MacLaren. 1962. Presence in the human placenta and term serum of a highly lactogenic substance immunologically related to pituitary growth hormone. Endocrinology 71:209–220.

Kalkhoff, R. K., D. S. Schalch, J. L. Walker, P. Beck, D. M. Kipnis, and W. H. Daughaday. 1964. Diabetogenic factors associated with pregnancy. Trans. Assoc. Am. Physicians 77:270–280.

Kane, J. E. 1973. A rapid electrophoretic technique for identification of subunit species of apoproteins in serum lipoproteins. Anal. Biochem. 53:350–364.

Karsznia, R., and H. Kaffarnik. 1969. Untersuchungen der serumlipide während schwanger-shaft und wochenbett. Arch. Gynaekol. 207:505–512.

Kessler, G., and H. Lederer. 1965. Fluorometric measurement of triglycerides, pp. 341–344. *In* Automation in Analytical Chemistry. Technicon Symposia. Mediad, Inc., White Plains, N.Y.

King, K. C., J. Butt, K. Raivio, N. Räihä, J. Roux, K. Teramo, K. Yamaguchi, and R. Schwartz. 1971. Human maternal and fetal insulin response to arginine. N. Engl. J. Med. 285:607–612.

Knopp, R. H., E. Herrera, and N. Freinkel. 1970. Carbohydrate metabolism in pregnancy. VIII. Metabolism of adipose tissue isolated from fed and fasted pregnant rats during late gestation. J. Clin. Invest. 49:1438–1446.

Knopp, R. H., M. R. Warth, and C. J. Carrol. 1973a. Lipid metabolism in pregnancy. I. Changes in lipoprotein triglyceride and cholesterol in normal pregnancy and the effects of diabetes mellitus. J. Reprod. Med. 10:95–101.

Knopp, R. H., C. D. Saudek, R. A. Arky, and J. B. O'Sullivan. 1973b. Two phases of adipose tissue metabolism in pregnancy: maternal adaptations for fetal growth. Endocrinology 92:984–988.

Knopp, R. H., M. Boroush, and J. B. O'Sullivan. 1975. Lipid metabolism in pregnancy. II. Postheparin lipolytic activity and hypertriglyceridemia in the pregnant rat. Metabolism 24:481–493.

Konttinen, A. T., Pyörälä, and E. Carpén. 1964. Serum lipid pattern in normal pregnancy and pre-eclampsia. J. Obstet. Gynaecol. Br. Commonw. 71:453–458.

Kühl, C. and J. J. Holst. 1976. Plasma glucagon and insulin: glucagon ratio in gestational diabetes. Diabetes 25:16–23.

Leon, L., R. L. Rush, and J. Turrell. 1970. Automated simultaneous cholesterol and triglyceride determination on the autoanalyzer II instrument, pp. 503–507, *In* Advances in Automated Analysis. Technicon International Congress, vol. I, Clinical Analysis. Mediad, Inc., White Plains, N.Y.

Lind, T., and F. E. Hytten. 1972. The excretion of glucose during normal pregnancy. J. Obstet. Gynaecol. Br. Commonw. 79:961–965.

Lind, T., H. A. Van C. de Groot, G. Brown, and G. A. Cheyne. 1972. Observations on blood glucose and insulin determinations. Br. Med. J. 3:320–323.

Lind, T., W. Z. Billewicz, and G. Brown. 1973. A serial study of changes occurring in the oral glucose tolerance test in pregnancy. J. Obstet. Gynaecol. Br. Commonw. 80:1033–1039.

Lipid Research Clinics Program. 1974. Manual of Laboratory Operations. National Heart and Lung Institute, Bethesda, Md. DHEW Publication No. NIH-75-628. 103 pp.

Litchfield, C., 1972. Analysis of Triglycerides. Academic Press, Inc., New York. 355 pp.

Lofland, H. B., Jr. 1964. A semi-automated procedure for the determination of triglycerides in serum. Anal. Biochem. 9:393–400.

Lott, J. A., and K. Turner. 1975. Evaluation of Trinder's glucose oxidase method for measuring glucose in serum and urine. Clin. Chem. 21:1754–1760.

Lunell, N. O., B. Persson, and G. Ohgvist. 1973. The effects of an oral combined contraceptive on plasma levels of glucose, free fatty acids, glycerol, D-β-hydroxybutyrate and triglycerides. Acta Obstet. Gynecol. Scand. 52:23–24.

Luyckx, A. S., J. Gerard, U. Gaspard, and P. J. Lefebvre. 1975. Plasma glucagon levels in normal women during pregnancy. Diabetologia 11:549–554.

Mager, M., and G. Farese. 1965. What is "true" blood glucose? Am. J. Clin. Pathol. 41:104–108.

McDonald-Gibson, R. G., M. Young, and F. E. Hytten. 1975. Changes in plasma nonesterified fatty acids and serum glycerol in pregnancy. Br. J. Obstet. Gynaecol. 82:460–466.

Montes, A., J. J. Albers, and R. H. Knopp. 1976. Contrasting apolipoprotein changes in pregnancy and lactation. Program of the 58th Annual Meeting of the Endocrine Society (June 23–25). Abstract No. 255.

Oliver, M. F., and G. S. Boyd. 1955. Plasma lipid and serum lipoprotein patterns during pregnancy and postpartum. Clin. Sci. 14:15–23.

O'Sullivan, J. B. 1970. Gestational diabetes and its significance, pp. 339–346. *In* R. A. Camerini-Davalos, ed., Early Diabetes. Academic Press, Inc., New York.

O'Sullivan, J. B., and N. Kantor. 1963. Variability of blood sugar levels with an automated method. Public Health Rep. 78:1023–1029.

O'Sullivan, J. B., and C. M. Mahan. 1964. Criteria for the oral glucose tolerance test in pregnancy. Diabetes 13:278–285.

O'Sullivan, J. B., and C. M. Mahan. 1966. Glucose tolerance test. Variability in pregnant and nonpregnant women. Am. J. Clin. Nutr. 19:345–351.

O'Sullivan, J. B., and G. W. McDonald. 1966. Decisive factors in designing the Sudbury study of chronic disease. Public Health Rep. 81:891–897.

O'Sullivan, J. B., S. S. Gellis, R. V. Dandrow, and B. O. Tenney. 1966. The potential diabetic and her treatment in pregnancy. Obstet. Gynecol. 27:683–689.

O'Sullivan, J. B., P. J. Snyder, A. C. Sporer, R. V. Dandrow, Jr., and D. Charles. 1970. Intravenous glucose tolerance test and its modification by pregnancy. J. Clin. Endocrinol. Metab. 31:33–37.

O'Sullivan, J. B., C. M. Mahan, D. Charles, and R. V. Dandrow. 1973. Screening criteria for high-risk gestational diabetic patients. Am. J. Obstet. Gynecol. 116:895–900.

O'Sullivan, J. B., C. M. Mahan, D. Charles, and R. V. Dandrow. 1974a. Medical treatment of the gestational diabetic. Obstet. Gynecol. 43:817–821.

O'Sullivan, J. B., C. M. Mahan, R. B. D'Agostino, and D. Charles. 1974b. Glucose disposal rates and the glucose challenge in pregnant women. J. Clin. Endocrinol. Metab. 39:1067–1071.

O'Sullivan, J. B., L. Aiello, E. Carrington, J. J. Hoet, R. H. Knopp, and R. Schwartz. 1975. Report of the workgroup on pregnancy of the Committee on Scope and Impact, pp. 177–244. *In* Report of the National Commission on Diabetes to the Congress of the United States, vol. III, part 2. U.S. Government Printing Office, Washington, D.C. Publication No. HEW-NIH-76-1022.

Pedersen, J. 1967. The Pregnant Diabetic and Her Newborn. Williams and Wilkins Co., Baltimore. 219 pp.

Persson, B., and N. O. Lunell. 1975. Metabolic control in diabetic pregnancy. Variations in plasma concentrations of glucose, free fatty acids, glycerol, ketone bodies, insulin, and human chorionic somatomammotropin during the last trimester. Am. J. Obstet. Gynecol. 122:737–745.

Peters, J. P., M. Heineman, and E. B. Man. 1951. Lipids of serum in pregnancy. J. Clin. Invest. 30:388–394.

Picard, C., H. A. Ooms, E. Balasse, and V. Conard. 1968. Effect of normal pregnancy on glucose assimilation, insulin and nonesterified fatty acids levels. Diabetologia 4:16–19.

Rappaport, F., and F. Eichorn. 1960. Sulfosalicylic acid as a substitute for paratoluene sulfonic acid. Clin. Chim. Acta 5:161–163.

Romano, A. T. 1973. Automated glucose methods: evaluation of a glucose oxidase-peroxidase procedure. Clin. Chem. 19:1152–1157.

Russ, M., H. A. Eder, and D. P. Barr. 1954. Protein-lipid relationships in human plasma. III. In pregnancy and the newborn. J. Clin. Invest. 33:1662–1669.

Sabata, V., H. Wolf, and S. Lausman. 1968. The role of free fatty acids, glycerol, ketone bodies and glucose in the energy metabolism of the mother and fetus during delivery. Biol. Neonate 13:7–17.

Samaan, N., S. C. C. Yen, H. Friesen, and O. H. Pearson. 1966. Serum placental lactogen levels during pregnancy and in trophoblastic disease. J. Clin. Endocrinol. Metab. 26:1303–1308.

Samsioe, G., P. Johnson, and A. Gustafson. 1975. Studies in normal pregnancy. I. Serum lipids and fatty acid composition of serum phosphoglycerides. Acta Obstet. Gynecol. Scand. 54:265–270.

Saudek, C. D., M. Finkowski, and R. H. Knopp. 1975. Plasma glucagon and insulin in rat pregnancy: roles in glucose homeostasis. J. Clin. Invest. 55:180–187.

Schonfeld, G., and B. Pfleger. 1974. The structure of human high density lipoprotein and the levels of apoprotein Al in plasma as determined by radioimmunoassay. J. Clin. Invest. 54:236–246.

Seltzer, H. S. 1970. Diagnosis of diabetes, pp. 436–507. *In* M. Ellenberg and H. Rifkin, eds., Diabetes Mellitus: Theory and Practice, 2nd ed. McGraw-Hill Book Co., New York.

Silverstone, F. A., E. Solomons, and J. Rubricius. 1961. The rapid intravenous glucose tolerance test in pregnancy. J. Clin. Invest. 40:2180–2189.

Skipper, E. 1933. Diabetes mellitus and pregnancy. A clinical and analytical study. Q. J. Med. 2:353–380.

Soler, N. G., and J. M. Malins. 1971. Prevalence of glycosuria in normal pregnancy. A quantitative study. Lancet I:619–621.

Spellacy, W. N., and F. C. Goetz. 1963. Plasma insulin in normal late pregnancy. N. Engl. J. Med. 268:988–991.

Spellacy, W. N., F. C. Goetz, B. Z. Greenberg, and J. Ells. 1965a. Plasma insulin in normal "early" pregnancy. Obstet. Gynecol. 25:862–865.

Spellacy, W. N., F. C. Goetz, B. Z. Greenberg, and J. Ells. 1965b. Plasma insulin in normal midpregnancy. Am. J. Obstet. Gynecol. 92:11–15.

Spellacy, W. N., F. C. Goetz, B. E. Greenberg, and K. L. Schoeller. 1965c. Tolbutamide response in normal pregnancy. J. Clin. Endocrinol. Metab. 25:1251–1254.

Statland, B. E., H. Bakelund, and P. Winkel. 1974. Factors contributing to intra-individual variation of serum constituents. 4. Effects of posture and tourniquit application on variation of serum constituents in healthy subjects. Clin. Chem. 20:1513–1519.

Sunderman, F. W., Jr., and F. W. Sunderman. 1961. Measurement of glucose in blood, serum, and plasma by means of a glucose oxidase-catalase enzyme system. Am. J. Clin. Pathol. 36:75–91.

Sutherland, H. W., and J. M. Stowers. 1975. The detection of chemical diabetes during pregnancy using the intravenous glucose tolerance test, pp. 153–166. *In* H. W. Sutherland and J. M. Stowers, eds., Carbohydrate Metabolism in Pregnancy and The Newborn. Churchill Livingstone, New York.

Sutherland, H. W., J. M. Stowers, and C. McKenzie. 1970. Simplifying the clinical problem of glycosuria in pregnancy. Lancet I:1068–1071.

Svanborg, A., and O. Vikrot. 1965. Plasma lipid fractions, including individual phospholipids at various stages of pregnancy. Acta Med. Scand. 178:615–630.

Tan, M. H., E. G. Wilmshurat, R. E. Gleason, and J. S. Soeldner. 1973. Effect of posture on serum lipids. N. Engl. J. Med. 289:416–419.

Taylor, G. O. 1972. Serum lipids and fatty acid composition in pregnant Nigerian women. J. Obstet. Gynaecol. Br. Commonw. 29:68–71.

Taylor, G. O., and E. O. Akande. 1975. Serum lipids in pregnancy and socioeconomic status. Br. J. Obstet. Gynaecol. 82:297–302.

Technicon Autoanalyzer Method File No. 24. 1972. Simultaneous cholesterol/triglycerides, pp. 1–6. Technicon Instruments Corp.

Tonks, D. B. 1967. The estimation of cholesterol in serum: a classification and critical review of methods. Clin. Biochem. 1:12–29.

Tyson, J. E., and T. J. Merimee. 1970. Some physiologic effects of protein ingestion in pregnancy. Am. J. Obstet. Gynecol. 107:797–800.

Tyson, J. E., D. Rabinowitz, T. J. Merimee, and H. Friesen. 1969. Response of plasma insulin and human growth hormone to arginine in pregnant and postpartum females. Am. J. Obstet. Gynecol. 103:313–319.

Van Handel, E., and D. B. Zilversmit. 1957. Micromethod for the direct determination of serum triglycerides. J. Lab. Clin. Med. 50:152–157.

Varma, S. K., P. H. Sonksen, K. Varma, J. S. Soeldner, H. A. Selenkow, and K. Emerson, Jr. 1971. Measurement of human growth hormone in pregnancy and correlation with human placental lactogen. J. Clin. Endocrinol. Metab. 32:328–332.

Victor, A. 1974. Normal blood sugar variation during pregnancy. Acta Obstet. Gynecol. Scand. 53:37–40.

Von Studnitz, W. 1955. Studies on serum lipids and lipoproteins in pregnancy. Scand. J. Clin. Lab. Invest. 7:329–335.

Wahlefeld, A., S. Klose, and E. Munz. 1975. Fully enzymatic triglyceride determination (UV) in serum—a single channel method for the AAII- and SMA-autoanalyzer. Clin. Chem. 21:942. (Abstr.)

Warth, M. R., and R. H. Knopp. 1977. Lipid metabolism in pregnancy. V. Interactions of diabetes, body weight, age, and high carbohydrate diet. Diabetes 26:1056–1062.

Warth, M. R., R. A. Arky, and R. H. Knopp. 1975. Lipid metabolism in pregnancy. III. Altered lipid composition in intermediate, very low, low, and high density lipoprotein fractions. J. Clin. Endocrinol. Metab. 41:649–655.

Watson, W. C. 1957. Serum lipids in pregnancy and the pueperium. Clin. Sci. 16:475–480.

WHO Expert Committee. 1965. Diabetes Mellitus. World Health Organization Technical Report Series, No. 310. 30 pp.

Wieland, O. 1963. Glycerol, pp. 211–214. *In* H. U. Bergmeyer, ed., Methods of Enzymatic Analysis. Academic Press, Inc., New York.

Wilkerson, H. L. C., and J. B. O'Sullivan. 1963. A study of glucose tolerance and screening criteria in 752 unselected pregnancies. Diabetes 12:313–318.

Wybenga, D. R., and J. A. Inkpen. 1974. Lipids, pp. 1421–1493. *In* R. J. Henry, D. C. Cannon, and J. W. Winkleman, eds., Clinical Chemistry Principles and Techniques, 2nd ed. Harper and Row, New York.

Yen, S. S. C., P. Vela, and C. C. Tsai. 1970. Impairment of growth hormone secretion in response to hypoglycemia during early and late pregnancy. J. Clin. Endocrinol. Metab. 31:29–32.

Yen, S. S. C., C. C. Tsai, and P. Vela. 1971. Gestational diabetogenesis: quantitative analysis of glucose-insulin interrelationships between normal pregnancy and pregnancy with gestational diabetes. Am. J. Obstet. Gynecol. III:792–800.

Zalme, E., and H. C. Knowles, Jr. 1965. A plea for plasma sugar. Diabetes 14:165–166.

Zlatkis, A., B. Zak, and A. Boyle. 1953. A new method for the direct determination of serum cholesterol. J. Lab. Clin. Med. 41:486–492.

5

Nitrogenous Indices

ROY W. BONSNES

CREATININE

Serum

Serum creatinine is determined with or without the use of Lloyd's reagent. Serum creatinine levels of normal adult nonpregnant women range from 0.5–1.0 mg/dl when Lloyd's reagent is used (Henry et al., 1974) and from 0.8–1.2 mg/dl without Lloyd's reagent.

Sims and Krantz (1958) and Kuhlbäck and Widholm (1966) report the serum creatinine level during the second and third trimesters of pregnancy to be lower than in the nonpregnant state. Although Kuhlbäck and Widholm found the serum creatinine level during the first trimester to be similar to the nonpregnant level, Sims and Krantz (1958), on the basis of limited data from four patients, reported that the creatinine level during the first trimester decreased to essentially the level maintained throughout the rest of pregnancy. Kuhlbäck and Widholm did not use Lloyd's reagent, while Sims and Krantz did (see Table 5-1). Considering the difference in methodology, the agreement between the two reports is reasonably good.

Subsequently, Lind et al. (1971), using a method employing Lloyd's reagent, found creatinine levels during the last trimester to be only slightly lower than that expected in the nonpregnant state, i.e., an

89

TABLE 5-1 Serum Creatinine (mg/dl ± SD) Levels during Pregnancy

References	No. Patients	Nonpregnant	Trimester		
			1	2	3
Kuhlbäck et al. (1966)[a]	-, 30, 26, 25	0.83 ± 0.16	0.73 ± 0.11	0.58 ± 0.18	0.53 ± 0.16
Sims and Krantz (1958)	16, 4, 16, 32	0.67 ± 0.07	0.43 ± 0.02	0.47 ± 0.07	0.48 ± 0.07
Lind et al. (1971)	-, 28, 43, 138	–	(0.55 ± 0.10)[b]	(0.60 ± 0.11)[c]	0.64 ± 0.11[d]

[a]Cross-sectional study.
[b]6 to 20 wk.
[c]30 wk or less.
[d]31 through 39 wk and over. Presented by weeks in the original report; averaged here.

90

average of 0.63, with a range of from 0.38 to 0.89 mg/dl. This level is about 1.14 times higher than the average (about 0.56) reported by Kuhlbäck and Widholm and about 1.32 times the average value (about 0.48) reported by Sims and Krantz for the third trimester of pregnancy. Creatinine levels early in pregnancy may be slightly lower than during the third trimester (Lind *et al.*, 1971). These data are summarized in Table 5-1.

The differences are most probably due to differences in the procedures used for determination of serum creatinine since the analysis of serum is technically difficult, particularly with low levels of serum creatinine.

Urine

The creatinine excreted in the urine has been used classically to determine the completeness of the collection of a 24-h urine. The validity of the basic concept is questionable (Vestergaard and Leverett, 1958; Chattaway *et al.*, 1969). The extent of the variation is indicated in a recent longitudinal study in which 182 24-h urines collected biweekly from 20 normal patients from wk 21 through 40 of pregnancy were analyzed for creatinine by the Folin (1917) method (Aubrey *et al.*, 1975). The average 24-h excretion of creatinine for the whole group was 1.13 ± 0.15 g, and the coefficient of variation was 13 percent. Similar results were obtained for three normal pregnant patients from whom 24-h urines were collected daily during the third trimester until they delivered (Bonsnes *et al.*, 1963). Creatinine clearance is variable and can be diminished by a diet low in creatine, for example (Calloway and Margen, 1971).

Creatinine Clearance

The creatinine clearance of the normal adult nonpregnant woman ranges between 82–146 mg/min/1.73 m² (Henry *et al.*, 1974). There has been much controversy concerning the significance and interpretation of the creatinine clearance in the human. The present prevalent acceptance of the endogenous creatinine clearance as a measure of glomerular filtration rate seems to date back to a report by Brod and Sirota (1948). Data on the creatinine clearance during pregnancy by Sims and Krantz (1958) and by Bucht (1951) as summarized by the authors are presented in Table 5-2.

Generally, the values presented by Bucht are higher than those of Sims and Krantz. Most striking are those for the nonpregnant controls.

TABLE 5-2   Creatinine Clearance

References	No. of Patients	Mean (ml/min)	SD
Bucht (1951)			
2–8[a]	19	186.0	51.5
9–10	13	153.0	23.6
Nonpregnant	22	148.0	21.0
Sims and Krantz (1958)			
3[a]	3	171.0	15.53
4	3	194.0	6.55
5	7	164.3	21.38
6	4	163.8	40.42
7	7	160.9	27.38
8	10	161.4	32.61
9	7	159.7	27.69
10	11	142.7	29.00
Puerperium	3	102.7	17.79
Nonpregnant	17	101.0	23.05

[a]Lunar month.

Bucht's average value of 148 ml/min is 46 percent higher than that of Sims and Krantz. Moreover, Bucht's value is higher and that of Sims and Krantz is lower than might be expected if endogenous creatinine clearance approximates glomerular filtration rate as measured by inulin. The average of the two values (125 mg/min) is likely an acceptable value for the glomerular filtration rate of the normal nonpregnant woman.

Differences in methodology probably account for the variance in reported data.

UREA

Blood, Serum, and Plasma

The serum urea nitrogen of the normal adult human is reported by Henry et al. (1974) to be between 8–26 mg/dl. This range is probably too high for both pregnant and nonpregnant women. A more accurate range for clinically normal adult women is from 6–18 mg/dl (Bonsnes, 1948). Plasma values are essentially the same as serum values; whole-blood values (BUN) are 92 to 93 percent lower, depending upon the hematocrit.

The concentration of urea and thus urea nitrogen in the blood in any individual changes with the state of hydration, the metabolic rate, kidney function, and protein intake. In normal-pregnancy hydration, anabolic rate and kidney function increase. These changes result in a decrease in blood urea nitrogen. Protein intake, if adequate, is the only factor that tends to increase the urea nitrogen.

That blood urea nitrogen is reduced during pregnancy was first reported by Folin in 1917. This report has been adequately substantiated by three different groups of investigators using different methods (Table 5-3). The small differences observed are most likely due to differences in methodology, or diet of the populations studied.

Urine

The total nitrogen excreted in the urine per day is a function of protein intake. In turn, the urea excreted in the urine is a function of total nitrogen excreted. On a normal diet resulting in the excretion of about 11 g of total nitrogen per day, about 85 percent is urea nitrogen (Beard, 1935). On a high-protein diet, with about 15 g of total nitrogen in the urine per day, approximately the same percentage of the urea nitrogen is excreted (Folin, 1905; Beard, 1935). However, when protein intake is low, urinary total nitrogen falls, and urea nitrogen accounts for a decreasing percentage of total nitrogen. For example, when urinary total nitrogen is about 8.0 g, urea nitrogen accounts for 77–80 percent of total nitrogen (Folin, 1905; Beard, 1935); at about 5 g of total urinary nitrogen per day, urea nitrogen accounts for about 60 percent of the total nitrogen (Folin, 1905). At extremely low levels of nitrogen intake (about 1.6 g per day), urea nitrogen excretion is only 20 percent (Smith, 1926).

This general pattern of excretion of total nitrogen probably holds for the pregnant women, though it may be somewhat altered in magnitude. Certainly, it holds at the higher levels of protein intake.

For example, 24-h urine samples from three patients receiving a diet containing approximately 75 g of protein (12 g of nitrogen) a day were analyzed for total nitrogen by the micro-Kjeldahl method (Parnas and Wagner, 1921; Oser, 1965) and urea nitrogen by the single-channel Autoanalyzer (Bonsnes *et al.*, 1963). Between 86–88 percent of total nitrogen excreted per day was urea nitrogen. The coefficients of variation were under 2.2 percent, a figure lower than the coefficient of variation for the daily total urea nitrogen excretion. The excretion of urea nitrogen in relation to total nitrogen correlates well with protein nutrition in the pregnant patient (Beydoun *et al.*, 1972).

TABLE 5-3 Whole Blood or Serum Urea Nitrogen (mg/dl, ± sD) during Pregnancy

References	No. Patients	Nonpregnant	Trimester		
			1	2	3
Bonsnes (1948)[a] (whole blood)	29, 36, 28, 8	10.79 ± 2.77	7.14 ± 1.67	7.00 ± 1.95	8.05 ± 2.08
Sims and Krantz (1958) (serum)	21, –, 14, 32	12.50 ± 2.71	9.38 ± 1.39	9.38 ± 1.70	8.35 ± 0.43
Lind et al. (1971) (serum)	–, 35, 43, 144	–	(8.40 ± 2.24)[b]	(7.90 ± 2.60)[c]	8.12 ± 1.83[d]

[a]Cross-sectional study.
[b]6 to 20 wk.
[c]30 wk or less.
[d]31 through 39 wk and over. Presented by weeks in original report: averaged here.

Urea Clearance

Maximal urea clearance values (C_m—with urine flow of 2 ml/min or more) range between 59–95 ml/min/1.73 m²; standard clearances (C_s—urine flow of less than 2 ml/min) range between 20–65 ml/min/m² (Henry *et al.*, 1974). In order to make the maximal and standard clearances roughly comparable, it is possible to use the factor 75 as the average normal C_m and 54 for the average normal so that data can be expressed as percent of normal.

Urea clearance during pregnancy has been measured by many investigators. Reports vary considerably, and urea clearance has been observed to be decreased, normal, or elevated in pregnancy. The observations by Bonsnes and Lange (1950) and of Bucht (1951) that the inulin clearance is markedly increased throughout most of pregnancy, but may decrease near term, suggest that urea clearance likely is elevated during normal pregnancy.

Table 5-4 includes data of Horwitz and Ohler (1932) and that collected by Bonsnes (1948) on patients who might possibly have had a change in renal function. At the time and place the latter data were collected, urea clearances of from 100–170 percent of nonpregnant clearances were considered normal for pregnancy.

These data are of interest because the clearances were carried out as routine procedures. At about the same time, however, an investigation of the urea clearance throughout pregnancy yielded a value of 135 percent of normal with a standard deviation of 16. This lower standard deviation (16 versus approximately 23) is due to the fact that many fewer people were involved in carrying out the clearances.

TABLE 5-4   Urea Clearance in Pregnancy

References	No. Patients	Mean (% of Nonpregnant)	SD
Horwitz and Ohler (1932)			
(trimester not stated)	9	136.0	28.11
Bonsnes (unpublished data)			
1st Trimester	36	129.6	21.35
2nd Trimester	27	134.7	25.10
3rd Trimester	4	125.0	17.45
Nonpregnant	28	98.2	12.97

URIC ACID

Serum Uric Acid

Serum uric acid levels of normal nonpregnant females range from 2.5–6.8 mg/dl when a uricase method is used and from 2.8–7.5 mg/dl when a phosphotungstate method is used (Henry et al., 1974).

Data from the literature on serum uric acid during pregnancy are shown in Table 5-5. Steenstrup (1956) and Sample et al. (1974) used uricase methods. Both investigators report low values early in pregnancy with an upward trend throughout pregnancy; values are generally below those observed in the nonpregnant state. Dash and Verma (1969) and Boyle et al. (1966), using phosphotungstate methods, observed relatively constant values throughout pregnancy, which were in the lower range for the normal adult nonpregnant females. Considering the differences in the methods used these data agree fairly well. The decrease in serum uric acid is likely due to the increased glomerular filtration rate that accompanies pregnancy.

Urine Uric Acid

Only one study on uric acid excretion during normal pregnancy has been reported (Boyle et al., 1966). The amount excreted during the first trimester is essentially the same as that excreted in the nonpregnant state, about 600 mg/24 h. However, in the second and third trimesters, significantly higher amounts are excreted, about 925 mg/24 h in the second trimester and about 830 mg/24 h in the third trimester.

ENZYMES

Alkaline Phosphatase

The alkaline phosphatase level in the normal nonpregnant adult female ranges from 4–17 King-Armstrong units (Henry et al., 1974), 1.5–4.0 Bodansky units (Bodansky, 1933), or 30–85 mU/ml on the Technicon SMA 12/60.

Serum alkaline phosphatase increases progressively as pregnancy progresses (Table 5-6). This increase appears to be due to the secretion of a heat-stable alkaline phosphatase (HSAP) by the placenta. Pregnancy also is accompanied by an increase in alkaline phosphatase from tissues other than the placenta, since the HSAP remains constant over time at about 70 percent of the total alkaline phosphatase (TAP).

TABLE 5-5 Serum Uric Acid (mg/dl ± SD) Levels during Pregnancy

References	No. Patients	Nonpregnant	Trimester			Months			
			1	2	3	2–3	4–5	6–7	8–9
Boyle et al. (1966)	64, 44, 48, 14	3.86 ± 0.72	2.72 ± 0.62	2.60 ± 0.54	2.61 ± 0.75				
Sample et al. (1974)	26, 13, 13, 13	4.36 ± 0.77	3.02 ± 0.61	3.19 ± 0.61	3.86 ± 0.61				
Steenstrup (1956)	45, 93, 43, 15, 90	3.70 ± 0.95				2.95 ± 0.55	2.94 ± 0.53	3.05 ± 0.50	3.60 ± 0.75
Dash and Verma (1969)	98, 20, 14, 12, 27	2.78 ± 0.28				2.64 ± 0.94	2.29 ± 0.88	2.36 ± 0.34	2.64 ± 1.32

TABLE 5-6 Alkaline Phosphatase

Week of Pregnancy	Aleem (1972) (King-Armstrong Units)			Elder (1972) (PIU)[a]		Bagga et al. (1969) (Bodansky Units)	
	No.	Total	Heat Stable	No.	Heat Stable	No.	Total
8	—					2	1.66
12–16	—					11	2.15 ± 0.89
17–24	—					8	6.44 ± 3.8
25	—						
26	6	8.61 ± 1.77	5.24 ± 1.04			10	8.10 ± 4.9
27	—						
28	11	9.74 ± 2.02	6.60 ± 1.72	14	11.7 ± 3.31		
29	5	9.84 ± 1.19	7.54 ± 0.89				
30	14	10.76 ± 2.45	7.75 ± 1.53	9	11.0 ± 4.98	13	11.62 ± 6.9
31	8	11.83 ± 2.26	8.73 ± 1.53	17	13.3 ± 4.96		
32	11	12.60 ± 2.31	8.67 ± 1.96	17	12.8 ± 4.99		
33	9	12.31 ± 1.34	8.93 ± 1.65	17	13.8 ± 6.21		
34	18	14.28 ± 3.04	10.07 ± 3.27	27	16.6 ± 6.80	11	15.32 ± 6.59
35	15	14.13 ± 3.13	10.34 ± 2.00	23	17.5 ± 5.87		
36	20	15.35 ± 3.81	10.14 ± 2.72	30	17.5 ± 4.95		
37	26	16.50 ± 3.25	10.90 ± 2.31	37	19.2 ± 5.91		
38	27	17.22 ± 2.11	12.41 ± 2.34	30	20.0 ± 6.04		
39	23	18.41 ± 3.50	13.07 ± 3.29	24	20.9 ± 5.64		
40	12	19.95 ± 3.46	13.37 ± 3.05	16	19.1 ± 6.73		
41	7	21.65	15.80	9	19.3 ± 5.26		
42				7	20.3 ± 8.52		
40–42				32	19.4 ± 6.58		

[a]PIU = placental isoenzyme units (see Elder, 1972).

98

It is difficult to compare enzyme values of different investigators because the activity expressed as units varies with substrate concentration, temperature and other factors. It is possible, however, to compare the ratios of activities.

For example, Aleem (1972) reported both TAP and HSAP in King-Armstrong units from wk 26 onward. The HSAP activity during 14 wk reported averaged about 70 percent of the TAP, while the TAP increased about 2.3 times during this time. This number is close to the other coefficients of variation presented. Bagga *et al.* (1969) also found that the HSAP was 70 percent of the TAP during gestation. If approximately 70 percent of the serum TAP is HSAP of placental origin, the increase in TAP during pregnancy is partially derived from other tissues as well.

Aspartate Amino Transferase, Alanine Amino Transferase, Lactic Dehydrogenase

Most reports of the serum levels of aspartate amino transferase and alanine amino transferase agree that they remain within nonpregnant limits throughout pregnancy regardless of the method of assay or the units used. There may well be a slight continuous rise well within the normal range throughout pregnancy.

Some investigators have reported elevations of serum lactic dehydrogenase (LD) levels in otherwise normal pregnancies. Unless it is known that the serum has been separated from the red cells shortly after the blood has been drawn, it might be better to consider the elevation of the LD to be due to LD from red blood cells, since red cells contain approximately 160 times as much LD as serum. It seems likely that the pattern of serum LD throughout pregnancy is much like that of the amino transferases.

Table 5-7 contains the data of Romalis and Claman (1962), which is

TABLE 5-7 Aspartate Amino Transferase, Alanine Amino Transferase, and Lactic Dehydrogenase Levels in Normal Pregnancy[a]

Week of Pregnancy	AST			ALT			LD		
	No.	Mean	Range	No.	Mean	Range	No.	Mean	Range
1–14 wk	18	7.9	3–14	17	5.1	1–12	18	88.2	62–123
15–28 wk	41	9.3	3–20	39	5.6	1–17	41	91.4	55–133
28–40 wk	65	11.1	2–46	61	6.9	1–20	65	92.6	58–146

[a]From Romalis and Claman (1962).

representative of the slight increase in serum levels during pregnancy
of these three enzymes.

AMINO ACIDS

The α-amino nitrogen in plasma is lower during pregnancy than in the
nonpregnant state (Bonsnes and Brew, 1947; Macdonald and Good,
1971). As shown in Figure 5-1, it is lowest early in pregnancy, increases
somewhat in midpregnancy, and then decreases again near term (Macdonald and Good, 1971).

It has been known for some time that the excretion of certain amino
acids is increased during pregnancy. For example, the increase in the
histidine concentration in the urine has been used as a pregnancy test
(Voge, 1929).

Plasma levels of 19 individual amino acids (Hytten and Cheyne,
1972) are presented in Table 5-8. Levels of most plasma amino acids
are lower during pregnancy than those found 8 wk postpartum. There
is, however, considerable variation. The plasma level of arginine may
increase up to wk 20 of pregnancy, but then decreases to below the

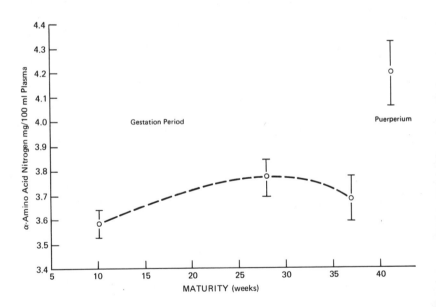

FIGURE 5-1   Plasma amino nitrogen concentrations during pregnancy and the early
puerperium. From Macdonald and Good (1971).

TABLE 5-8   Plasma Amino Acids during Pregnancy[a]

Amino Acid	Under 20 wk	20–29 wk	30 wk and Over	8 wk Postpartum
Alanine	295 ± 56	338 ± 69	341 ± 89	382 ± 128
Arginine	80 ± 24	68 ± 31	59 ± 23	75 ± 33
Asparagine	28 ± 9	28 ± 13	27 ± 13	32 ± 23
Cystine	22 ± 9	37 ± 24	24 ± 11	33 ± 21
Glutamic acid	145 ± 56	148 ± 79	167 ± 64	162 ± 71
Glycine	161 ± 37	154 ± 37	132 ± 44	246 ± 105
Histidine	92 ± 22	92 ± 11	93 ± 17	92 ± 34
Isoleucine	58 ± 19	50 ± 15	49 ± 11	56 ± 23
Leucine	100 ± 27	99 ± 20	85 ± 18	105 ± 46
Lysine	163 ± 41	170 ± 31	152 ± 26	212 ± 99
Methionine	12 ± 8	13 ± 7	12 ± 5	18 ± 15
Ornithine	46 ± 10	53 ± 13	46 ± 15	93 ± 43
Phenylalanine	54 ± 18	56 ± 13	50 ± 9	61 ± 24
Proline	150 ± 58	151 ± 62	167 ± 51	251 ± 88
Serine	135 ± 50	143 ± 62	118 ± 44	169 ± 73
Taurine	80 ± 34	75 ± 26	62 ± 15	104 ± 69
Threonine	295 ± 46	378 ± 75	354 ± 106	400 ± 118
Tyrosine	47 ± 18	42 ± 6	45 ± 6	68 ± 31
Valine	186 ± 45	178 ± 33	156 ± 33	204 ± 93

[a]Plasma amino-acid concentrations (μmol/l) in pregnancy and in the postpartum period from ten normal subjects (mean ± SD) from Hytten and Cheyne, 1972.

nonpregnant level. The plasma level of histidine is unchanged during pregnancy.

Urinary excretion rates of the individual amino acids are generally increased during pregnancy over what is observed 8 wk postpartum, although there is considerable variation. The specific reasons for the fall in the plasma levels and the large increase in the urinary excretion of the amino acids are not known. Plasma concentrations of amino acids vary during the menstrual cycle and are decreased in women on oral contraceptives (Craft and Peters, 1971). This finding suggests a role of steroid hormones in regulating plasma amino acid levels.

SERUM PROTEINS

Total Serum Proteins and Albumin

The total serum proteins of the normal adult range between 6.6–8.3 g/dl; for albumin, 3.5–5.0 g/dl; for α_1-globulin, 0.1–0.4 g/dl; for α_2-

globulin, 0.6–1.2 g/dl; and for gamma globulin, 0.5–1.5 g/dl (Henry *et al.*, 1974).

Using classical chemical methods, it is well documented that the total protein of serum gradually decreases during pregnancy. At about wk 28, it levels off, after which it remains essentially constant (Table 5-9). The fall in serum total protein is due largely to the decrease in the serum albumin (Table 5-10), which, as Macdonald and Good (1971) have pointed out, falls more than the total protein because of the elevation of some of the globulin fractions.

Serum Globulins

The globulins of serum can be separated by free and paper electrophoresis. These fractions migrate more slowly than albumin and in order are called α_1, α_2, β and gamma globulins. The majority of reports agree that there is a small increase in the α_1, α_2, and β globulins in pregnancy, with a decrease in the gamma globulins, but with no change during the course of pregnancy (Hytten and Lind, 1973). Illustrative of paper electrophoretic patterns of pregnancy sera is Table 5-11 from MacGillivray and Tovey (1957).

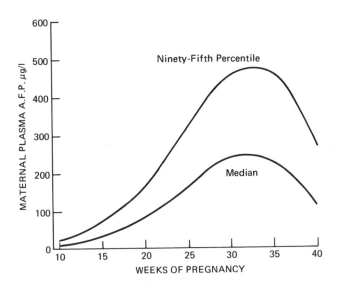

FIGURE 5-2 Median and ninety-fifth percentile of maternal plasma-AFP throughout normal pregnancy. From Leighton *et al.* (1975).

TABLE 5-9 Serum Total Protein in Pregnancy[a]

References	Type of Study	No. of Subjects	Method of Estimation	Serum Total Protein (g/100 ml) at wk of Pregnancy:									
				Non-pregnant	4–8	9–12	13–16	17–20	21–24	25–28	29–32	33–36	37–40
Von Studnitz (1955)	Cross-sectional	101	Kjehldahl	7.1	7.1	7.0	6.8	6.6	6.6	6.5	6.6	6.6	6.8
MacGillivray and Tovey (1957)	Partly longitudinal	13	Kjehldahl	7.3			7.3		6.8	6.6		6.6	
De Alvarez et al. (1961)	Partly longitudinal	28	Biuret	7.18	7.27	6.61	5.62	5.59	5.74	5.96	6.01	5.74	5.90
Reboud et al. (1967)	Cross-sectional	135	Densimetric	7.03		6.73	6.68	6.14	6.33	5.94	6.27	6.13	6.13
Kruglov (1967)	Longitudinal	103	Refraction	8.09	7.33	7.23	7.00	6.88	6.91	6.94	6.96	7.07	7.20
Wilken and Schwebke (1968)	Longitudinal	75	Biuret	No data		7.13			6.76		6.74		6.72
Robertson (1969) and personal communication	Longitudinal	83	Biuret	7.04		6.47	6.36	6.29		6.26	6.23	6.19	6.24

[a]Published with permission of Blackwell Scientific Publications Ltd., Oxford, England. From F. E. Hytten and I. Leitch, *The Physiology of Human Pregnancy*, 2nd ed., 1971, p. 49.

TABLE 5-10   Serum Albumin in Pregnancy[a]

References	Type of Study	No. of Subjects	Method	Serum Albumin (g/100 ml) at wk of Pregnancy:									
				Non-pregnant	4–8	9–12	13–16	17–20	21–24	25–28	29–32	33–36	37–40
Von Studnitz (1955)	Cross-sectional	101	Paper electrophoresis	4.53	4.36	4.43	4.18	3.95	3.79	3.74	3.69	3.52	3.69
MacGillivray and Tovey (1957)	Partly longitudinal	13	Paper electrophoresis	4.63		4.20		3.91		3.34		3.34	
De Alvarez et al. (1961)	Partly longitudinal	28	Paper electrophoresis	3.62	3.69	3.12	2.57	2.62	2.67	2.75	2.72	2.45	2.40
Reboud et al. (1967)	Cross-sectional	135	Paper electrophoresis	3.33		3.13	2.87	2.53	2.59	2.33	2.38	2.30	2.38
Kruglov (1967)	Longitudinal	103	Paper electrophoresis	4.48	3.88	3.69	3.53	3.42	3.38	3.33	3.30	3.30	3.33
Wilken and Schwebke (1968)	Longitudinal	75	Paper electrophoresis	No data		4.87			4.33		4.24		4.00
Robertson (1969) and personal communication	Longitudinal	83	Paper electrophoresis,	3.42		3.22	3.04	2.93		2.81	2.80	2.75	2.75
			Chemical precipitation	4.04		3.83	3.67	3.60		3.46	3.45	3.44	3.42

[a]Published with permission of Blackwell Scientific Publications Ltd., Oxford, England. From F. E. Hytten and I. Leitch, *The Physiology of Human Pregnancy*, 2nd ed., 1971, p. 49.

TABLE 5-11   Serum Protein Changes in Pregnancy[a]

| Protein | Normal Nonpregnant Values | | Normal Pregnancy | | | | | | | |
| | | | 8–16 wk | | 16–24 wk | | 23–32 wk | | 32–40 wk | |
	gm/dl ± SD	% of Total	gm/dl	% of Total	gm/dl	% of Total	gm/dl	% of Total	gm/dl	% of Total
Albumin	4.63 ± 0.33	66.8 ± 4.7	4.20	60.7	3.91	61.0	3.34	53.6	3.34	54.7
α_1-Globulin	0.24 ± 0.06	2.9 ± 0.9	0.29	3.6	0.32	4.2	0.35	4.9	0.39	5.4
α_2-Globulin	0.52 ± 0.10	6.4 ± 1.4	0.65	8.2	0.65	8.6	0.78	10.7	0.77	10.7
β-Globulin	0.93 ± 0.11	10.3 ± 1.6	1.01	11.7	0.95	11.8	1.21	15.8	1.25	15.8
γ-Globulin	0.98 ± 0.21	13.7 ± 3.0	1.15	15.8	0.97	14.6	0.92	15.0	0.85	13.4
Total Protein	7.3	7.3	7.3	7.3	6.8	6.8	6.6	6.6	6.6	6.6
No. of Cases	100	100	13	13	13	13	15	15	13	13

[a]From MacGillivray and Tovey (1957).

α_1-Fetoprotein

α_1-Fetoprotein (AFP) is synthesized by the fetal liver and yolk sac (Gitlin and Boesman, 1967). It increases in fetal serum from wk 6 to its highest concentration at about wk 13 of gestation, and thereafter it decreases to low levels by wk 34 (Gitlin and Boesman, 1966).

Bruck and Sutcliffe (1972) hypothesized that abnormally high levels of α_1-fetoprotein in amniotic fluid could permit detection of a fetus with anencephaly or spina bifida early in pregnancy. Since then, there have been many reports on measuring AFP in amniotic fluid as a marker for neural tube defects. But, amniocentesis, as an invasive technique, has certain drawbacks for screening purposes.

More recently, a simple, rapid radioimmunoassay has permitted the determination of AFP in maternal serum for screening purposes (Leek *et al.*, 1975). Leighton *et al.* (1975) prospectively screened 1,322 pregnant women for AFP levels in normal pregnancy (Figure 5-2).

REFERENCES

Aleem, F. A. 1972. Total and heat-stable serum alkaline phosphatase in normal and abnormal pregnancies. Obstet. Gynecol. 40:163–172.

Aubry, R. H., J. E. Rouke, V. G. Cuenca, and L. D. Marshall. 1975. Random urine estrogen/creatinine ration. A practical and reliable index of fetal welfare. Obstet. Gynecol. 46:64–68.

Bagga, O. P., V. D. Mullick, P. Madan, and S. Dewan. 1969. Total serum alkaline phosphate and its isoenzymes in normal and toxemic pregnancies. Am. J. Obstet. Gynecol. 104:850–855.

Beard, H. H. 1935. Coefficients of correlation between the nitrogenous constituents of urine after ingestion of low, normal and high protein diets. Hum. Biol. 7:419–429.

Beydoun, S. N., V. G. Cuenca, L. P. Evans, and R. H. Aubry. 1972. Maternal Nutrition. Am. J. Obstet. Gynecol. 114:198–203.

Bodansky, A. 1933. Phosphatase studies. II. Determination of serum phosphatase factors influencing the accuracy of the determination. J. Biol. Chem. 101:93–104.

Bonsnes, R. W. 1948. Unpublished data.

Bonsnes, R. W., and E. M. Brew. 1947. The plasma amino acid and amino nitrogen concentration during normal pregnancy, labor and early puerperium. J. Biol. Chem. 168:345–350.

Bonsnes, R. W., and W. A. Lange. 1950. On the inulin clearance during pregnancy. Fed. Proc. 9:154.

Bonsnes, R. W., M. Platt, and A. Marney. 1963. Unpublished data.

Boyle, J. A., S. Campbell, A. M. Duncan, W. R. Creig, and W. W. Buchanan. 1966. Serum uric acid levels in normal pregnancy with observations on the renal excretion of urate in pregnancy. J. Clin. Pathol. 19:501–503.

Brod, J., and J. Sirota. 1948. The renal clearance of endogenous "creatinine" in man. J. Clin. Invest. 27:645–654.

Bruck, D. J. H., and R. G. Sutcliffe. 1972. Alpha-fetoprotein in the antenatal diagnosis of anencephaly and spina bifida. Lancet ii:197–199.

Bucht, H. 1951. Studies on renal function in man. Scand. J. Clin. Lab. Invest. 3(Suppl. 3):1–64.

Calloway, D. H., and S. Margen. 1971. Variation in endogenous nitrogen excretion and dietary nitrogen utilization as determinants of human protein requirement. J. Nutr. 101:205–216.

Chattaway, F. W., R. P. Hullin, and F. C. Odds. 1969. Variability of creatinine excretion in normal subjects, mental patients and pregnant women. Clin. Chim. Acta 26:267–276.

Craft, I. L., and T. J. Peters. 1971. Quantitative changes in plasma amino acids induced by oral contraceptives. Clin. Sci. 41:301–307.

Dash, S., and S. N. Verma. 1969. Blood uric acid level in pregnancy. J. Indian Med. Assoc. 53:585–587.

Elder, M. G. 1972. Serum heat-stable alkaline phosphatase levels in normal and abnormal pregnancy. Am. J. Obstet. Gynecol. 113:833–837.

Folin, O. 1905. A theory of protein metabolism. Am. J. Physiol. 13:117–138.

Folin, O. 1917. Recent biochemical investigations on blood and urine; their bearing on clinical and experimental medicine. J. Am. Med. Assoc. 69:1209–1214.

Gitlin, D., and M. Boesman. 1966. Serum α-fetoprotein, albumin and γ-globulin in the human conceptus. J. Clin. Invest. 45:1836–1839.

Gitlin, D., and M. Boesman. 1967. Sites of serum α-fetoprotein synthesis in the human and in the rat. J. Clin. Invest. 46:1010–1016.

Henry, R. J., D. C. Cannon, and J. W. Winkelman. 1974. Clinical Chemistry: Principles and Technics. Harper & Row, Publishers, New York. (Front and back inside covers)

Horwitz, D., and W. R. Ohler. 1932. The urea clearance test in toxemias of pregnancy. J. Clin. Invest. 11:1119–1128.

Hytten, F. E., and G. A. Cheyne. 1972. The aminoaciduria of pregnancy. J. Obstet. Gynaecol. Br. Commonw. 79:424–432.

Hytten, F. E., and T. Lind. 1973. Diagnostic Indices in Pregnancy. Ciba-Geigy Corp., Basel, Switzerland. 122 pp.

Kulbäck, B., and O. Widholm. 1966. Plasma creatinine in normal pregnancy. Scand. J. Clin. Lab. Invest. 18:654–656.

Leek, A. E., C. F. Ruoss, M. J. Kitau, and T. Chard. 1975. Maternal plasma alpha-fetoprotein levels in the second half of normal pregnancy: relationship to fetal weight and maternal age and parity. Br. J. Obstet. Gynaecol. 82:669–673.

Leighton, P. C., Y. B. Gordon, J. M. Kitau, A. F. Leek, and T. Chard. 1975. Levels of alpha-fetoprotein in maternal blood as a screening test for fetal neural-tube defect. Lancet 2:1012–1015.

Lind, T., W. Z. Billewicz, and G. A. Cheyne. 1971. Composition of amniotic fluid and maternal blood through pregnancy. J. Obstet. Gynaecol. Br. Commonw. 78:505–512.

Macdonald, H. N., and W. Good. 1971. Changes in plasma total proteins, albumin, urea and alpha-amino nitrogen concentrations in pregnancy and the puerperium. J. Obstet. Gynaecol. Br. Commonw. 78:912–917.

MacGillivray, I., and J. E. Tovey. 1957. A study of the serum protein changes in pregnancy and toxemia using paper strip electrophoresis. J. Obstet. Gynaecol. Br. Commonw. 64:361–364.

Oser, B. L. 1965. Hawk's Physiological Chemistry, 14th ed. The Blakiston Division, McGraw-Hill. New York. 1219 pp.

Parnas, J. K., and R. Wagner. 1921. Ueber die Ausführung von Bestimmungen kleiner Stickstoffmengen nach Kjeldahl. Biochem. Z. 125:253–256.

Romalis, G., and A. D. Claman. 1962. Serum enzymes in pregnancy. Am. J. Obstet. Gynecol. 84:1104–1110.

Sample, P. F., W. Carswell, and J. A. Boyle. 1974. Serial studies of the renal clearance of urate and inulin during pregnancy. Clin. Sci. Mol. Med. 47:559–565.

Sims, E. A. H., and K. Krantz. 1958. Serial studies on renal function during normal pregnancy and the puerperium in normal women. J. Clin. Invest. 37:1764–1774.

Smith, M. 1926. The minimum endogenous nitrogen metabolism. J. Biol. Chem. 68:15–31.

Steenstrup, O. R. 1956. Hypouricemia during pregnancy. Scand. J. Clin. Lab. Invest. 8:263–264.

Vestergaard, P., and R. Leverett. 1958. Constancy of urinary creatinine excretion. J. Lab. Clin. Med. 51:211–218.

Voge, C. 1929. A simple chemical test for pregnancy. Br. Med. ii:829–830.

6

Vitamin
Indices

HOWERDE E. SAUBERLICH

Various biochemical methods have been developed over the past 25 yr that have proved useful in the evaluation of the nutritional status for most vitamins. The techniques are based on measurement of several indices including: (a) changes in enzyme activities on blood components that can be related to intake of a given vitamin, (b) abnormal metabolic products in blood or urine resulting from a deficient or submarginal intake of a given vitamin, (c) level of a given vitamin in blood or urine, (d) urinary metabolites of a given vitamin, and (e) saturation or load tests of a given vitamin.

In general, these biochemical measurements can provide an objective assessment of the nutritional status of an individual with respect to specific vitamins. However, as will be noted, for some of the procedures only limited experience is available concerning their usefulness in evaluating nutritional status during pregnancy. In some instances, values are available only for nonpregnant adult subjects. Undoubtedly, as the biochemical procedures become increasingly available and employed, more precise indices applicable during pregnancy will evolve.

In view of the various methods employed in individual laboratories for measuring a given vitamin, caution must be exercised in the utilization of the values presented. Moreover, the vitamin levels observed may be influenced by numerous factors including maternal age, multivitamin intake, season of the year, parity, social class, smoking,

109

previous use of oral contraceptive agents, intake of medicinal agents, and fetal sex. The values presented are representative of the information available and may provide guidance for the establishment of normal values during pregnancy.

VITAMIN A

Conflicting reports exist as to serum vitamin A changes accompanying pregnancy. Darby *et al.* (1953b) observed that serum vitamin A levels fell about 10 percent during pregnancy and then rose again postpartum. These investigators regarded the decreased serum levels during pregnancy as reflecting a normal phenomenon, perhaps related to pregnancy-associated changes in lipid metabolism (Darby *et al.*, 1948). Similar observations were reported by Pulliam *et al.* (1962). On the other hand, Lewis *et al.* (1974) reported that the decline in blood vitamin A values during the last trimester could be prevented with daily supplements of retinol or carotene, suggesting that the decrease in serum vitamin A reflects increased demands during pregnancy.

In more recent studies, al-Nagdy *et al.* (1971) found no significant difference in serum vitamin A levels in pregnant and nonpregnant women. Morse *et al.* (1975) also found no change in plasma vitamin A levels over time in pregnancy but did observe a significant increase postpartum. Gal and Parkinson (1972, 1974) reported, however, a decrease in serum vitamin A levels in the first trimester, followed by an increasing trend as pregnancy advanced. Toward the end of pregnancy, vitamin A levels again decreased, but rose following delivery, returning almost to nonpregnant levels by 6 wk postpartum. In contrast, Basu and Arulanantham (1973) observed a decrease in serum retinol levels in subjects with a low socioeconomic background as pregnancy advanced to full term.

Serum vitamin A levels of lactating women have been observed to be higher than those of the women not breast-feeding their infants (Gal and Parkinson, 1972, 1974). Although the magnitude of these changes in serum vitamin A in the normal subject is relatively small, these variations should be kept in mind when conducting and interpreting vitamin A studies in lactation (Gal and Parkinson, 1974).

The state of vitamin A nutriture of the mother is reflected in the level of the vitamin in the breast milk and in liver stores of the infant at birth as a result of placental transfer (al-Nagdy *et al.*, 1971; Rodriguez and Irwin, 1972). Prolonged low intakes of vitamin A are usually reflected in low serum levels of retinol.

Vitamin A is transported in the plasma by a specific retinol-binding protein (Glover, 1973; Underwood, 1974). The levels of plasma retinol-binding protein correlate closely with plasma retinol levels. Serum and plasma vitamin A may be readily measured with the use of colorimetric, spectrophotometric, or fluorometric procedures (Thompson *et al.*, 1973; Sauberlich *et al.*, 1974).

Laboratory indices for vitamin A nutritional status in the adult female are given in Table 6-1.

VITAMIN C (ASCORBIC ACID)

The measurement of serum levels of ascorbic acid is the most commonly used and practical procedure for determining vitamin C nutritional status (Sauberlich *et al.*, 1974; Sauberlich, 1975). Although leukocyte and whole-blood ascorbate levels have been measured in human subjects, little information is available concerning levels during pregnancy.

Serum vitamin C levels have been observed to decrease 10–15 percent during pregnancy (Darby *et al.*, 1953b; Vobecky *et al.*, 1974a; Morse *et al.*, 1975). These changes have been suggested as indicating an increased requirement for vitamin C as pregnancy advances (Vobecky *et al.*, 1974a). However, in view of the reported effects of the phase of the menstrual cycle and of ingestion of oral contraceptive agents on the ascorbic-acid levels in plasma and leukocytes, these decreases may be related in part to hormonal adjustments occurring during pregnancy (McLeroy and Schendel, 1973; Rivers, 1975). Darby *et al.* (1953a, 1953b) observed a further decrease in serum ascorbic acid levels during postpartum, especially in lactating women. Morse *et al.* (1975), however, did not observe a significant change in plasma ascorbic acid during the postpartum period.

Ascorbic acid can be measured in serum or plasma with the use of automated or manual colorimetric and fluorometric procedures (Sauberlich *et al.*, 1974, 1976; Sauberlich, 1975).

Laboratory indices for vitamin C nutritional status in the adult female are given in Table 6-2.

THIAMIN

Various biochemical techniques have been developed that have been useful for assessing thiamin nutrition status (Sauberlich *et al.*, 1974). The most commonly used procedure has been the measurement by

TABLE 6-1 Biochemical Assessment of Vitamin A Nutritional Status in the Adult Female

Test	Special Conditions	Display	Non-pregnant	Pregnancy Trimester 1	Pregnancy Trimester 2	Pregnancy Trimester 3	Post-partum	References
Serum or plasma retinol (µg/dl)		Mean ± SD	25 ± 10 (11)[a]	–	36 ± 8 (11)	32 ± 17 (34)	30 ± 13 (8)	Garcia et al. (1974)
		Mean ± SD	–	33 ± 9 (332)	33 ± 9 (686)	29 ± 9 (553)	43 ± 11 (1,493)	Darby et al. (1953b)
		Mean ± SE	–	50 ± 3.1 (57)	50 ± 2.4 (95)	50 ± 2.5 (168)	62 ± 2.6 (89)	Morse et al. (1975)
		Mean ± SD	–	25.6 ± 7.6 (2,793)	24.0 ± 7.8 (1,883)	24.6 ± 9.3 (204)	35.3 ± 8.9 (128)	Edozien et al. (1976)
		Mean ± SE	26 ± 1.0 (278)	33 ± 0.6 (344)	34 ± 0.3 (1,086)	30 ± 0.3 (699)	–	Darby et al. (1953a)
		Mean ± SD	38 ± 8 (21)	–	–	22 ± 5 (25)	30 ± 8 (15)	Pulliam et al. (1962)
		Mean ± SD	38 ± 8 (348)	–	–	–	–	Sauberlich (1976a)
		Range	20–68	–	–	–	–	Health Services and Mental Health Administration (1972)
		Mean	55 (6,563)	–	–	–	–	

	Statistic						Reference
Low-income subjects	Mean ± SE	31 ± 2 (12)	30 ± 2 (10)	24 ± 1 (24)	23 ± 1 (56)	—	Basu and Arulanantham (1973)
	Mean ± SD	52 ± 11 (24)	—	—	51 ± 15 (36)	—	al-Nagdy et al. (1971)
	Range	25–78			22–78		
	Mean ± SD	42 ± 8 (30)	25 ± 14 (30)	40 ± 34 (30)	57 ± 28 (30)	47 ± 21 (30)	Gal and Parkinson (1972, 1974)
	Mean ± SE	52 ± 0.76 (2,406)	—	—	—	—	U.S. Department of Health, Education, and Welfare (1974)
Adolescents	Mean	—	73 (26)	47 (81)	40 (129)	—	McGanity et al. (1969)
No OCA[b]	Mean ± SD	37 ± 1.9 (32)	—	—	33 ± 1.7 (22)	53 ± 31 (11)	Horwitt et al. (1975)
+ OCA	Mean ± SD	53 ± 2.5 (15)	—	—	—	—	
	Range	28–83					
No OCA	Mean ± SD	44 ± 10 (80)	—	—	—	—	Smith et al. (1975)
+ OCA	Mean ± SD	54 ± 12 (84)	—	—	—	—	Smith et al. (1975)

[a] Values in parentheses indicate number of subjects studied.
[b] Oral contraceptive agents.

113

TABLE 6-2 Biochemical Assessment of Vitamin C Nutritional Status in the Adult Female

Test	Special Conditions	Display	Non-pregnant	Pregnancy Trimester 1	Pregnancy Trimester 2	Pregnancy Trimester 3	Post-partum	References
Serum vitamin C (mg/dl)		Mean ± SD	0.95 ± 0.46 (16)[a]	—	1.25 ± 0.30 (11)	0.97 ± 0.38 (34)	0.67 ± 0.33 (10)	Garcia et al. (1974)
		Median	0.50 (125)	0.45 (195)	0.39 (287)	0.34 (399)	0.20 (1,140)	Darby et al. (1953b)
		Mean ± SD Range	0.58 ± 0.32 (348) 0.08 – 1.48	—	—	—	—	Sauberlich (1976a)
		Mean ± SE	—	1.43 ± 0.06 (58)	1.37 ± 0.05 (94)	1.10 ± 0.05 (76)	1.10 ± 0.05 (90)	Morse et al. (1975)
		Mean ± SE	0.98 ± 0.04 (106)	—	—	—	—	Darby et al. (1953a)
		Mean ± SD	—	0.60 ± 0.22 (229)	0.66 ± 0.24 (475)	0.54 ± 0.25 (922)	—	Vobecky et al. (1974a)
	High-income states	Mean	0.87 (1,776)	—	—	—	—	Health Services and Mental Health Administration (1972)
	Low-income states	Mean	0.58 (470)	—	—	—	—	Health Services and Mental Health Administration (1972)

114

							Reference
No OCA[b]	Mean ± SE	0.63 ± 0.05 (32)	—	—	1.22 ± 0.11 (22)	0.74 ± 0.08 (11)	Horwitt et al. (1975)
+OCA	Mean ± SE	0.75 ± 0.08 (15)	—	—	—	—	Horwitt et al. (1975)
No OCA	Mean ± SD	0.39 ± 0.22 (84)	—	—	—	—	Smith et al. (1975)
+OCA	Mean ± SD	0.38 ± 0.22 (84)	—	—	—	—	Smith et al. (1975)
Nonsmokers	Mean ± SE	0.97 ± 0.05 (50)	—	—	—	—	Brook and Grimshaw (1968)
Moderate smokers	Mean ± SE	0.74 ± 0.07 (28)	—	—	—	—	Brook and Grimshaw (1968)
	Mean ± SD	—	0.95 ± 0.49 (1,866)	0.91 ± 0.47 (1,371)	0.85 ± 0.42 (166)	0.90 ± 0.52 (105)	Edozien et al. (1976)
Leucocyte Vitamin C mg/dl cells — No OCA	Mean ± SD	25.7 ± 145 (63)	—	—	—	—	McLeroy and Schendel (1973)
+OCA	Mean ± SD	19.4 ± 6.6 (49)	—	—	—	—	McLeroy and Schendel (1973)
µg/10⁸ cells — Nonsmokers	Mean ± SE	30.7 ± 1.4 (50)	—	—	—	—	Brook and Grimshaw (1968)
Moderate smokers	Mean ± SE	25.6 ± 1.6 (28)	—	—	—	—	Brook and Grimshaw (1968)

[a] Values in parentheses indicate number of subjects studied.
[b] Oral contraceptive agents.

chemical or microbiological methods of urinary levels of thiamin. A reasonably close correlation exists between the development of a thiamin deficiency and the decreasing excretion of thiamin in the urine. The thiamin requirement of the adult human has been considered to be approximately 0.30 to 0.35 mg per 1,000 cal. When this intake is maintained, 40 to 90 μg of thiamin is excreted in the urine daily. A correlation between thiamin intake and the urinary excretion of thiamin per gram of creatinine has been observed. Consequently, as a matter of expedience, random urine samples may be obtained (preferably during a fasting state) and the thiamin content related to creatinine content.

Urinary thiamin levels fall during the second and third trimester of pregnancy, with the most pronounced effects during the third trimester (Darby et al., 1953b). The level of excretion returns to normal slowly postpartum. These observations may reflect increased metabolic requirements for thiamin during pregnancy (Tripathy, 1968; Migasena et al., 1974).

Erythrocyte transketolase measurement has been shown to be a more reliable and sensitive indicator of thiamin status than urinary determinations of thiamin (Sauberlich, 1967; Sauberlich et al., 1974). The erythrocyte transketolase stimulation represents any enhancement in enzyme activity, expressed in percent, resulting from the in vitro addition of thiamin pyrophosphate (Sauberlich et al., 1974). The measurement has been utilized to assess thiamin status in pregnancy (Tripathy, 1968; Chong and Ho, 1970; Heller et al., 1974; Migasena et al., 1974; Morse et al., 1975; Watson and Dako, 1975). Subjects with an erythrocyte transketolase stimulation of less than 15 percent are commonly considered normal or acceptable in terms of thiamin nutriture (Brin et al., 1965; Sauberlich et al., 1974). Automated analyzer systems have provided rapid, simple, sensitive, and reproducible assay methods.

Laboratory indices for thiamin nutritional status in the adult female are given in Table 6-3.

RIBOFLAVIN

The measurement of urinary excretion of riboflavin has been commonly used for evaluating the nutritional status of this vitamin (Darby et al., 1953b; Sauberlich et al., 1974). Correlations between dietary intakes of riboflavin and urinary excretions of the vitamin have been established through well-controlled human experiments. From these studies, guidelines for interpreting urinary riboflavin excretion data have been extrapolated.

During pregnancy, urinary excretion of riboflavin increases during the second trimester and falls during the third trimester (Darby *et al.*, 1953b). Normal excretion levels are observed postpartum. Although the significance of these changes is uncertain, guides have been developed to interpret urinary riboflavin excretion in pregnant women (Sauberlich *et al.*, 1974). These guidelines must be used with caution, however, because urinary riboflavin levels tend to reflect the recent dietary intake of the nutrient and, hence, are prone to considerable variation. The use of fasting urine samples helps reduce this effect. However, this effect is minimal in persons subsisting on marginal or inadequate intakes of riboflavin, whose body stores are depleted or unsaturated.

Erythrocyte glutathione reductase activity measurement represents a functional test of nutritional adequacy of riboflavin and largely avoids the limitations associated with urinary riboflavin excretion data. The measurement is simple and reproducible and requires only a minute quantity of blood (Nichoalds *et al.*, 1974). The assay results are usually expressed in terms of activity coefficients, representing the degree of stimulation resulting from the *in vitro* addition of flavin adenine dinucleotide (Nichoalds *et al.*, 1974; Sauberlich *et al.*, 1974). Activity coefficients for normal pregnant women appear to be comparable to normal nonpregnant subjects (Cooperman *et al.*, 1973; Iyengar, 1973; Nichoalds *et al.*, 1974).

The use of riboflavin load tests and the measurement of blood riboflavin levels have also been proposed to evaluate riboflavin nutritional status (Sauberlich *et al.*, 1974).

Laboratory indices for riboflavin nutritional status in the adult female are given in Table 6-4.

NIACIN (NICOTINIC ACID)

Biochemical procedures for evaluating niacin status are not entirely satisfactory, and few studies have been conducted on niacin nutritional status during pregnancy (Sauberlich *et al.*, 1974).

A functional biochemical test has not been developed for assessing body reserves of the nutrient. Nicotinic acid is present in only small amounts in the urine, and the excretion is relatively uninfluenced by dietary intakes of niacin or tryptophan. Little nicotinic acid is present in serum, but appreciable quantities are present in the leukocytes and erythrocytes as nicotinamide mononucleotide or dinucleotide. Thus far, however, measurement of niacin compounds in blood or its components has not appeared to be a reliable or satisfactory method for evaluating niacin status.

TABLE 6-3 Biochemical Assessment of Thiamin Nutritional Status in the Adult Female

Test	Special Conditions	Display	Nonpregnant	Pregnancy Trimester			Post-partum	References
				1	2	3		
Urinary thiamin excretion μg/2 h		Median	120 (61)[a]	130 (118)	100 (169)	70 (181)	90 (719)	Darby et al. (1953b)
μg/g of creatinine		Mean ± SD, Range	267 ± 146 (260) 49–914	–	–	–	–	Sauberlich (1976a)
	Male and female, age 17–34 yr	Mean	398 (1,432)	–	–	–	–	Health Services and Mental Health Administration (1972)
	Adolescents	Mean	–	200 (25)	220 (94)	225 (126)	–	McGanity et al. (1969)
Erythrocyte transketolase stimulation (%)		Mean ± SE	–	7.1 ± 0.6 (61)	6.2 ± 0.5 (99)	5.8 ± 0.5 (80)	5.6 ± 0.6 (96)	Morse et al. (1975)
	Low-income subjects	Mean ± SE	–	–	–	–	13 ± 5.8 (15)	Bamji (1976)
		Mean ± SD	5.6 ± 7.0 (344)	–	–	–	–	Sauberlich (1976a)
	7 females, 8 males	Mean	<15 (15)	–	–	–	–	Bayoumi and Rosalki (1976)

118

Measurement	Group	Statistic					Reference
	Age and sex unknown	Mean ± SD	11 ± 4.5 (10)	–	–	–	Smeets et al. (1971)
		Range	2–20				
	Adult male and female	Range	0–17 (39)	–	–	–	Massod et al. (1971)
		Mean ± SD	18 ± 26 (18)	–	–	–	Henshaw et al. (1970)
		Mean ± SD	–	13 ± 0.1 (41)	13 ± 0.1 (79)	13 ± 0.1 (171)	Heller et al. (1974)
	Indian women	Average	13 (14)	–	–	19 (16)	Bamji (1970)
	Ghanian women	Mean ± SD	24 ± 10 (42)	–	–	27 ± 9 (28)	Watson and Dako (1975)
	Malaysians	Mean ± SD	–	–	–	23 ± 15 (103)	Chong and Ho (1970)
Erythrocyte transketolase activity (IU) (μM/h/ml whole blood)							
Glycerol-3-PO_4 formation	7 females; 8 males	Mean	7.8 (15)[a]	–	–	–	Bayoumi and Rosalki (1976)
Glycerol-3-PO_4 formation	Age and sex unknown	Mean / Range	7.0 (10) / 5.0–9.2	–	–	–	Smeets et al. (1971)
Pentose disappearance	Adolescent females	Mean ± SD	11.96 ± 1.59 (178)	–	–	–	Warnock et al. (1975)

TABLE 6-3 (Continued)

Test	Special Conditions	Display	Nonpregnant	Pregnancy Trimester			Post-partum	References
				1	2	3		
Sedoheptulose-7-PO₄ formation		Mean ± SD	3.58 ± 0.65 (39)	—	—	—	—	
		Range	2.52–5.16					
	Adult male and female	Mean ± SD	2.13 ± 0.61 (42)	—	—	2.22 ± 0.59 (28)	—	Watson and Dako (1975)
		Mean ± SD	—	—	—	3.18 ± 0.84 (103)	—	Bayoumi and Rosalki (1976)

[a] Values in parentheses indicate number of subjects studied.

The two major metabolites of nicotinic acid are N^1-methyl-nicotinamide and N^1-methyl-2-pyridone-5-carboxylamide (2-pyridone) (Rosenthal *et al.*, 1953; Sauberlich *et al.*, 1974). The measurement of these metabolites in urine has been the usual means of assessing niacin status (Sauberlich *et al.*, 1974). The excretion of N^1-methyl-nicotinamide was observed to increase gradually during the second trimester of pregnancy and plateau during the third trimester (Sauberlich *et al.*, 1974). The level of excretion of the metabolite then rapidly returned to normal postpartum.

More recently, niacin status has been evaluated by the use of the 2-pyridone/N^1-methylnicotinamide excretion ratio (Joubert and De Lange, 1962; DeLange and Joubert, 1964; Sauberlich *et al.*, 1974). Under normal conditions, adults excrete 40 to 60 percent of their nicotinic acid as the 2-pyridone form and 20 to 30 percent as the N^1-methylnicotinamide form. With niacin deficiency, the urinary excretion of 2-pyridone is reduced more profoundly than that of N^1-methylnicotinamide. Thus, a ratio of 1.3 to 4 exists between 2-pyridone/N^1-methylnicotinamide excretion under normal conditions, while a ratio of less than 1.0 is indicative of a latent niacin deficiency. Although this appears to be the most practical index available for assessing niacin status, the procedure requires further evaluation with pregnant subjects to fully establish its reliability and usefulness.

Laboratory indices for niacin nutritional status in the adult female are given in Tables 6-5 and 6-6.

FOLIC ACID (FOLACIN)

Megaloblastic anemia resulting from folate deficiency occurs in a substantial proportion of pregnant women in developing countries and a smaller though still significant number of those in developed nations (Stone *et al.*, 1967; Rothman, 1970; Sauberlich *et al.*, 1974). Folacin nutritional status in the human has been assessed through procedures such as the assay of folate levels in serum, whole blood, erythrocytes, leukocytes, liver biopsy specimens, use of folacin loading tests, and measurement of urinary excretion of formiminoglutamic acid (FiGlu), urocanic acid, and aminoimidazolecarboxamide (AIC) (Herbert, 1965; Stone *et al.*, 1967; Sauberlich *et al.*, 1974). Of these procedures, measurement of serum folic acid levels is the most commonly performed. Nevertheless, serum folate level is probably a relatively poor indicator of the degree of folate deficiency (Hoffbrand *et al.*, 1966; Blakley, 1969) because low serum levels reflect recent low dietary intakes and provide little information concerning tissue reserves. Thus,

TABLE 6-4 Biochemical Assessment of Riboflavin Nutritional Status in the Adult Female

Test	Special Conditions	Display	Nonpregnant	Pregnancy trimester			Post-partum	References
				1	2	3		
Urinary riboflavin excretion								
mg/2 h		Mean ± SE	–	–	1.11 ± 0.04 (248)[a]	0.91 ± 0.03 (411)	0.88 ± 0.04 (340)	Darby et al. (1953a)
μg/g creatinine		Mean ± SD	481 ± 280 (259)	–	–	–	–	Sauberlich (1976a)
		Range	79–2,058					
		Mean	559 (839)					Health Services and Mental Health Administration (1972)
		Mean	–	230 (23)	220 (69)	200 (116)	–	McGanity et al. (1969)

122

Erythrocyte
glutathione
reductase
stimulation
(activity co-
efficients)[a]

			Various periods of time during pregnancy	Reference
	Mean ± SD	—	0.98 ± 0.05 (20)	Cooperman et al. (1973)
	Range	—	0.9–1.09	
Low-income subjects	Mean ± SE	—	1.69 ± 1.08 (15)	Bamji (1976)
	Mean ± SD	1.12 ± 0.13 (317)	—	Sauberlich (1976a)
Hospital patients	Mean	1.17 (8)	—	Bayoumi and Rosalki (1976)

[a]Values in parentheses indicate number of subjects studied.

123

TABLE 6-5   Biochemical Assessment of Niacin Nutritional Status
in the Adult Female[a]

Week Gestation or Postpartum	No. of Subjects	N[1]-methylnicotinamide Excretion (median values, mg/2h)
1st Trimester		
5–9	63	7.04
10–13	77	7.55
2d Trimester		
14–16	140	8.06
17–19	101	9.19
20–22	139	9.54
23–26	118	11.20
3d Trimester		
27–29	155	10.60
30–32	312	11.04
33–35	216	11.25
36 & over	53	10.62
Postpartum		
<6	57	
≥6	421	5.44

[a]From Darby et al. (1953b).

low serum folate levels are not necessarily associated with megaloblastic anemia or any biochemical changes (Herbert, 1965; Hoffbrand et
al., 1966; Blakley, 1969).

Folic acid is present in serum in association with serum folate-
binding proteins. Levels of serum folate-binding proteins may be
elevated in pregnancy and in women taking oral contraceptives
(Pritchard et al., 1971; Theuer, 1972; Shojania and Hornady, 1973).

Serum folate levels commonly fall during pregnancy, probably in
response to the marked increased demands for the vitamin, particularly
during the third trimester (Solomon et al., 1962; Kitay, 1969; Rothman,
1970; Iyengar, 1971; Sauberlich et al., 1974). A portion of the fall may
be due to the increased urinary excretion of folic acid reported to occur
in pregnancy (Landon and Hytten, 1971; Fleming, 1972). Administration of folic acid usually results in a prompt and significant increase in
serum folate values (Metz et al., 1965; Kitay, 1969; Iyengar, 1971).

The erythrocyte folate level has come to be regarded as a more
accurate and less variable quantitative index than serum folate as to the
severity of folacin deficiency (Herbert, 1965; Hoffbrand et al., 1966;
Kitay, 1969; Rothman, 1970; Sauberlich et al., 1974). Erythrocyte

TABLE 6-6 Biochemical Assessment of Niacin Nutritional Status in the Adult Female

Test	Display	Nonpregnant	Pregnancy Trimester			Post-partum	References
			1	2	3		
N¹-Methylnicotinamide excretion							
mg/g Creatinine	Mean (adult male & female)	4.3 (12)[a]	—	—	—	—	De Lange and Joubert (1964)
	Mean	—	8.5 (25)	9.6 (94)	10.2 (126)	—	McGanity et al. (1969)
μM/g Creatinine		26.1 ± 2.3 (32)	—	—	174 ± 28 (22)	30.3 ± 7.6 (11)	Horwitt et al. (1975)
mg/24 h	Range (men)	4.8–11.5 (10)	—	—	—	—	Joubert and De Lange (1962)
Urinary 2-pyridone excretion							
mg/g Creatinine	Mean (adult male & female)	8.7 (12)	—	—	—	—	De Lange and Joubert (1964)
mg/24 h	Mean (adult male & female)	2.1 (12)	—	—	—	—	De Lange and Joubert (1964)
	Range (men)	5.2–19.7 (10)	—	—	—	—	Joubert and De Lange (1962)

[a]Values in parentheses indicate number of subjects studied.

folate measurement has proven to be a useful biochemical test for evaluating folacin nutritional status in pregnancy (Chanarin et al., 1968; Kitay, 1969; Rothman, 1970; Colman et al., 1974; Colman et al., 1975; Hershko et al., 1975). Moreover, erythrocyte folate levels correlate well with response to folic acid supplementation (Metz et al., 1965; Chanarin et al., 1968; Balmelli and Huser, 1974; Colman et al., 1974, 1975; Hershko et al., 1975).

In evaluating folate levels in serum and erythrocytes, it must be recognized that the period of folate deficiency that will cause a drop in erythrocyte folate levels is much longer than that causing a decrease in the serum levels of folacin (Herbert, 1965; Kitay, 1969). In addition, it should be noted that erythrocyte folate measurements do not distinguish between megaloblastic anemia due to vitamin B_{12} deficiency and that due to a folacin deficiency. In subjects with a primary vitamin B_{12} deficiency, folic acid levels in the serum may be elevated while low levels may be encountered in the erythrocytes (Herbert, 1965; Nixon and Bertino, 1970; Sauberlich et al., 1974). However, a low folic acid value for both serum and erythrocytes is strong evidence that a folacin deficiency exists. Serum vitamin B_{12} measurements can be performed to eliminate further the possibility of pernicious anemia or of a dietary vitamin B_{12} deficiency.

Microbiological assay procedures have been used almost entirely to measure folacin levels in serum and erythrocytes, although isotopic assay procedures have been recently introduced (Sauberlich et al., 1974; Eichner et al., 1975).

Laboratory indices for folic acid nutritional status in the adult female are given in Table 6-7.

VITAMIN B_6

Because vitamin B_6 participates in a wide variety of enzyme reactions, numerous biochemical changes occur with a deficiency. Some of these changes have served as a means for detection of an inadequate dietary intake of the vitamin (Linkswiler, 1967; Sauberlich et al., 1970, 1972, 1974; Brown, 1972).

With a dietary restriction of vitamin B_6, man excretes increased amounts of xanthurenic acid, kynurenine, hydroxykynurenine, and other related metabolites following a tryptophan load test (Linkswiler, 1967; Leklem, 1971; Brown, 1972). Pregnant women may also excrete abnormal amounts of these metabolites (Brown et al., 1961; Wachstein, 1964; Hamfelt and Hahn, 1969; Rose and Braidman, 1971; Brown, 1972; Sauberlich and Canham, 1973). The abnormal excretions of tryptophan metabolites are reduced to normal or near normal levels with the administration of relatively large doses of pyridoxine (Rose and Braidman, 1971; Brown, 1972; Sauberlich and Canham, 1973). Of the tryptophan metabolites excreted in the urine, xanthurenic acid is the easiest to measure (Sauberlich *et al.*, 1970, 1972, 1974). Although the tryptophan load test is relatively easy to perform and has been widely used to evaluate vitamin B_6 status, the results of the test need to be interpreted with care in view of the interrelated metabolic and hormonal factors involved in tryptophan metabolism (Luhby *et al.*, 1971; Rose and Braidman, 1971; Brown, 1972). A methionine load test has also been used to evaluate vitamin B_6 status in pregnancy (Krishnaswamy, 1972). In vitamin B_6 deficiency, cystathionine excretion is markedly increased following a load of methionine.

The major urinary metabolite of vitamin B_6 is 4-pyridoxic acid. With inadequate intakes of the vitamin, the amount of 4-pyridoxic acid excreted is low or nil (Sauberlich *et al.*, 1972, 1974). The methods for measuring 4-pyridoxic acid in urine are rather tedious and involved and, hence, have seldom been used to evaluate vitamin B_6 nutritional status (Linkswiler, 1967; Contractor and Shane, 1970).

A number of studies have been conducted to ascertain the usefulness of measuring urinary levels of vitamin B_6 for evaluating the nutritional status of this nutrient (Sauberlich *et al.*, 1970, 1972, 1974). In controlled studies with adult subjects, the urinary excretion of free vitamin B_6 correlated closely with the level of intake of the vitamin. Urinary excretions of less than 20 μg/g of creatinine are indicative of marginal or inadequate dietary intakes of vitamin B_6 (Sauberlich *et al.*, 1972, 1974). However, little information is available concerning the urinary excretion of vitamin B_6 during pregnancy.

Vitamin B_6 levels in whole blood, erythrocytes, and plasma fall rapidly during vitamin B_6 depletion and rise following supplementation (Wachstein, 1964; Linkswiler, 1967; Baker and Frank, 1968; Hamfelt and Hahn, 1969; Hamfelt and Tuvemo, 1972; Sauberlich *et al.*, 1972, 1974; Sauberlich and Canham, 1973; Cleary *et al.*, 1975; Brophy and Siiteri, 1976). Levels of vitamin B_6 are at least twice as high in cord blood as in maternal blood (Contractor and Shane, 1970; Brin, 1971; Brophy and Siiteri, 1976). Improvements in the procedures used for measuring pyridoxal phosphate in serum and blood have led to the use of this index in evaluating vitamin B_6 status in human population groups (Hamfelt and Hahn, 1969; Chabner and Livingston, 1970; Hamfelt and Tuvemo, 1972; Cleary *et al.*, 1975; Brophy and Siiteri, 1976). Plasma levels of pyridoxal phosphate progressively decline during pregnancy; a daily supplement in excess of 2 mg is required to prevent the decline

TABLE 6-7 Biochemical Assessment of Folic Acid Nutritional Status in the Adult Female

Test	Special Conditions	Display	Nonpregnant	Pregnancy trimester 1	2	3	Post-partum	References
Serum of plasma folic acid (ng/ml)		Mean ± SD	5.5 ± 1.0 (15)[a]	–	–	–	–	Hall et al. (1975)
		Mean ± SD	4.7 ± 1.0 (16)	–	–	–	–	Hershko et al. (1975)
		Mean ± SD	8.2 ± 2.8 (348)	–	–	–	–	Sauberlich (1976c)
		Range	2.5–18.0					
		Mean	7.5 (3,181)	–	–	–	–	Sauberlich (1976c)
		Range	5–25	–	–	–	–	Rothman (1970)
		Mean	–	–	–	4.7	–	Solomon et al. (1962)
		Mean ± SE	–	6.3 ± 0.5 (19)	5.3 ± 0.5 (19)	4.3 ± 0.4 (18)	–	Hamfelt and Tuvemo (1972)
	Indian women	Mean ± SE	–	6.4 ± 0.6 (44)	4.9 ± 0.4 (72)	3.0 ± 0.4 (44)	–	Iyengar (1971)
		Mean	7.5 (20)	–	–	6.2 (85)	–	Avery and Ledger (1970)
		Mean	–	6.0 (57)	5.4 (57)	5.1 (57)	5.4 (57)	Metz et al. (1965)
		Mean ± SE	5.0 ± 0.29 (30)	4.6 (58)	3.3	2.7 ± 0.12 (132)	3.5 ± 0.22 (55)	Temperley et al. (1968)
	Chinese	Mean ± SD	–	–	–	4.5 ± 1.5 (331)	–	Hibbard and Hibbard (1972)

Group	Statistic						Reference
Malay	Mean ± SD	—	—	—	4.1 ± 1.1 (139)	—	Hibbard and Hibbard (1972)
Indian	Mean ± SD	—	—	—	3.3 ± 2.0 (73)	—	Hibbard and Hibbard (1972)
	Mean ± SD	—	—	—	3.4 ± 2.6 (54)	—	Landon and Oxley (1971)
No folate supplement	Mean	5–20	6.1 (101)	4.5 (101)	4.5 (101)	—	Chanarin et al. (1968)
200-μg/day folate supplement	Mean	—	6.6 (105)	6.7 (105)	6.3 (105)	—	Chanarin et al. (1968)
No OCA	Mean ± SD	5.4 ± 2.4 (71)	—	—	—	—	Smith et al. (1975)
+OCA	Mean ± SD	4.5 ± 2.0 (80)	—	—	—	—	Smith et al. (1975)
No OCA	Mean	8.1 (55)	—	—	—	—	Pritchard et al. (1971)
+OCA	Mean	8.0 (57)	—	—	—	—	Pritchard et al. (1971)
No OCA	Mean	6.3 (101)	—	—	—	—	Theuer (1972) Shojania and Hornady (1973)
+OCA	Mean	4.1 (162)	—	—	—	—	Theuer (1972) Shojania and Hornady (1973)
Erythrocyte folic acid (ng/ml)	Mean ± SD	250 ± 84 (15)	—	—	—	—	Hall et al. (1975)
	Mean	241 (2.404)	—	—	—	—	Sauberlich (1976c)

TABLE 6-7 (Continued)

Test	Special Conditions	Display	Nonpregnant	Pregnancy Trimester			Post-partum	References
				1	2	3		
	No folate supplement	Mean	165 (31)	157 (101)	139 (101)	118 (101)	—	Chanarin et al. (1968)
	200-μg/day folate	Mean	—	165 (105)	190 (105)	187 (105)	—	Chanarin et al. (1968)
		Mean ± SE	—	135 ± 9 (19)	161 ± 16 (19)	111 ± 10 (18)	—	Hamfelt and Tuvemo (1972)
	No folate supplement	Mean ± SE	—	—	145 ± 16 (26)	111 ± 12 (26)	113 ± 11 (26)	Iyengar (1971)
	200-μg/day supplemental folate	Mean ± SE	—	—	145 ± 12 (25)	185 ± 36 (25)	181 ± 16 (25)	Iyengar (1971)
	Chinese	Mean ± SD	—	—	—	219 ± 71 (331)	—	Hibbard and Hibbard (1972)
	Malay	Mean ± SD	—	—	—	219 ± 78 (139)	—	Hibbard and Hibbard (1972)
	Indian	Mean ± SD	—	—	—	167 ± 52 (73)	—	Hibbard and Hibbard (1972)
	No OCA	Mean ± SD	199 ± 62 (64)	—	—	—	—	Smith et al. (1975)
	+OCA	Mean ± SD	173 ± 57 (70)	—	—	—	—	Smith et al. (1975)

[a]Values in parentheses indicate number of subjects studied.

(Contractor and Shane, 1970; Hamfelt and Tuvemo, 1972; Reinken *et al.*, 1973; Cleary *et al.*, 1975; Shane and Contractor, 1975; Brophy and Siiteri, 1976).

Erythrocyte transaminase measurements represent a biochemical functional test that provides information regarding the state of deficiency or the degree of depletion of vitamin B_6 reserves (Linkswiler, 1967; Sauberlich *et al.*, 1970, 1972, 1974). Controlled human vitamin B_6 studies have demonstrated that erythrocyte aspartate aminotransferase (EGOT) and erythrocyte alanine aminotransferase (EGPT) activities fall with depletion of the vitamin (Raica and Sauberlich, 1965; Canham *et al.*, 1966). Erythrocyte transaminase activities provide a much closer reflection of vitamin B_6 status than serum transaminase activities. However, measurement of EGOT and EGPT activity, if combined with determination of the *in vitro* stimulation by pyridoxal phosphate, provides a better indication of vitamin B_6 status (Linkswiler, 1967; Sauberlich *et al.*, 1972, 1974). Erythrocytes contain considerably more GOT activity than that of GPT. Consequently, EGOT stimulation measurements are preferred over EGPT stimulation measurements in evaluating vitamin B_6 status during pregnancy (Hamfelt and Tuvemo, 1972; Reinken *et al.*, 1973; Shane and Contractor, 1975; Brophy and Siiteri, 1976). Considerable individual variation has been observed with normal individuals as to the erythrocyte transaminase activities either with or without the addition of pyridoxal phosphate. Part of this variation may be due to the analytical procedures employed. However, the EGOT stimulation in normal subjects is usually less than 60 percent, while a stimulation of over 100 percent may be encountered in vitamin-B_6-depleted subjects (Raica and Sauberlich, 1965; Canham *et al.*, 1966; Sauberlich *et al.*, 1972, 1974; Heller *et al.*, 1973). Additional studies are needed to establish the validity and usefulness of these guidelines in evaluating vitamin B_6 status in pregnancy.

Laboratory indices for vitamin B_6 nutritional status in the adult female are given in Table 6-8.

VITAMIN B_{12}

Vitamin B_{12} deficiency due to a lack of dietary intake of the nutrient is relatively rare, but may occur among vegan (vegetarians), who subsist exclusively on vegetables (Yusufji *et al.*, 1973; Sauberlich *et al.*, 1974). Most cases of vitamin B_{12} deficiency in the United States are the result of an impaired absorption of the vitamin due to lack of the intrinsic factor in the gastric secretions (pernicious anemia). The biochemical procedures employed to evaluate vitamin B_{12} status are designed to

TABLE 6-8 Biochemical Assessment of Vitamin B_6 Nutritional Status in the Adult Female

Test	Special Conditions	Display	Nonpregnant	Pregnancy Trimester			Post-partum	References
				1	2	3		
Urinary vitamin B_6 (μg/g creatinine)		Mean ± SD	40.5 ± 1.1 (1,370)[a]	—	—	—	—	Sauberlich (1976b)
		Mean ± SD	54.0 ± 23.0 (261)	—	—	—	—	Sauberlich et al. (1970)
		Range	14–147					Sauberlich (1976a)
Plasma pyridoxal phosphate (ng/ml)	2-2.5 mg B_6 supplement/day	Mean ± SD	10.5 ± 4.1	—	—	3.7 ± 1.5 (13)	—	Cleary et al. (1975); Lumeng et al. (1974)
	10 mg B_6 supplement/day	Mean ± SD	—	—	—	7.5 ± 4.5 (11)	—	Cleary et al. (1975)
		Average	8.4 ± 2.5 (20)	—	—	4.3 (19)	—	Wachstein et al. (1959)
		Range	5.2–12.0			2–8.6		
		Mean ± SE	—	6.2 ± 0.8 (19)	2.8 ± 0.6 (19)	1.4 ± 0.3 (18)	—	Hamfelt and Tuvemo (1972)
		Mean	16.9 (4)	—	—	4.3 (9)	—	Brophy and Siiteri (1976)

Measure	OCA	Statistic					Reference
Leucocyte pyridoxal phosphate (ng/million cells)	No OCA	Mean ± SD	12.1 ± 2.3 (23)	—	7.7 ± 3.7 (5)	—	Contractor and Shane (1970)
	+OCA	Mean ± SD	11.7 ± 3.2 (9)	—	—	—	Brown et al. (1975)
			9.15 ± 2.6 (15)				
	No OCA	Mean ± SD	9.4 ± 4.2 (77)	—	—	—	Lumeng et al. (1974)
	+OCA		7.8 ± 3.7 (55)				
	No OCA	Mean ± SD	9.6 ± 1.7 (12)	—	5.1 ± 1.3 (10)	—	Shane and Contractor (1975)
	+OCA		7.6 ± 1.1 (9)				
Urinary 4-pyridoxic acid μM/day		Mean	0.22 ± 0.05 (20)	—	0.09 (19)	—	Wachstein et al. (1959)
		Range	0.14–0.30		0.02–0.19		
		Mean ± SD	3.9 ± 0.7 (26)	—	—	—	Adams et al. (1976)
		Mean ± SD	3.0 ± 1.0 (24)	—	—	—	Brown et al. (1975)
mg/day		Mean ± SD	1.21 ± 0.84 (26)	—	1.45 ± 0.47 (10)	—	Contractor and Shane (1970)

TABLE 6-8 (Continued)

Test	Special Conditions	Display	Nonpregnant	Pregnancy Trimester 1	Pregnancy Trimester 2	Pregnancy Trimester 3	Post-partum	References
Xanthurenic acid excretion (after tryptophan load)								
μg/ml fasting morning urine		Mean	20.2 (6)	—	—	41.0 (7)	—	Sprince et al. (1951)
		Range	7.8–32.6	—	—	15.1–108.0	—	Wachstein and Gudaitis (1952)
mg/24 h		Mean	17 (10)	—	—	191 (14)	—	Wachstein and Gudaitis (1952)
		Range	4–30	—	—	63–324	—	Wachstein and Gudaitis (1953)
		Mean ± SE	—	—	254 (14)	198 ± 15 (86)	95 (9)	Brown et al. (1961)
		Range		—		170–813	—	
μM/24 h	No OCA	Mean ± SD	27.0 ± 8.0 (12)	—	—	—	—	Rose et al. (1975)

134

Measure	OCA	Statistic					Reference
	+OCA	Mean ± SD	426 ± 363 (9)	—	—	—	Adams et al. (1976)
		Mean	63.0 ± 40.0 (26)	—	—	—	Hamfelt and Tuvemo (1972)
μM/8 h	No OCA	Mean	193 (12)	—	—	—	Lumeng et al. (1974)
	+OCA	Mean ± SD	27.1 ± 5.7 (15)	—	—	—	Lumeng et al. (1974)
	No OCA	Range	38–500 (11)	—	—	—	Luhby et al. (1971)
	+OCA	Mean	<35 (10)	—	—	—	
			167 (33)	—	—	—	
μM/g Creatinine		Mean ± SE	54.0 ± 4.0 (32)	—	254 ± 82 (22)	72 ± 24 (11)	Horwitt et al. (1975)
Kynurenine excretion (after tryptophan load) μM/24 h		Mean ± SD	36.0 ± 20.0 (26)	183 (14)	—	—	Adams et al. (1976)
		Mean	29 (10)	—	—	133	Brown et al. (1961)

TABLE 6-8 (Continued)

Test	Special Conditions	Display	Nonpregnant	Pregnancy Trimester				References
				1	2	3	Post-partum	
Erythrocyte GOT stimulation (%)		Mean ± SD	69.0 ± 15.0 (26)	–	–	–	–	Adams et al. (1976)
	Low-income subjects	Mean ± SE	–	–	–	41.0 ± 7.0	–	Bamji (1976)
		Range	–	–	–	10.7–111.1	–	Cheney et al. (1965)
		Average	80 (7)					Lumeng et al. (1974)
	Hospital patients	Mean	72 (8)	–	–	–	–	Lumeng et al. (1974)
	7 Females; 8 males	Mean ± SD	83.0 ± 24.0 (15)	–	–	–	–	
		Mean ± SD	69.0 ± 17.0 (12)	–	–	68.0 ± 12.0 (10)	–	Shane and Contractor (1975)
		Mean ± SD	–	–	91.0 ± 16.0 (23)	116.0 ± 19.0 (23)	–	Reinken et al. (1973)
		Mean ± SD	53 (69)	64.0 ± 23.0 (40)	68.0 ± 31.0 (51)	64.0 ± 28.0 (142)	–	Heller et al. (1973)
		Mean ± SE	–	52.0 ± 8.0 (19)	61.0 ± 10.0 (19)	56.0 ± 6.0 (17)	–	Hamfelt and Tuvemo (1972)
	No OCA	Mean ± SD	77.0 ± 15.0 (30)	–	–	–	–	Rose et al. (1973)
	+OCA	Mean ± SD	71.0 ± 23.0 (65)	–	–	–	–	Rose et al. (1973)

Measurement	Statistic					Reference
Erythrocyte GPT stimulation (%)	Mean ± SD	19.0 ± 20.0 (26)	—	—	—	Adams et al. (1976)
	Average	25 (7)	—	—	—	Cheney et al. (1965)
	Range	0–15 (7)	—	—	—	Wachstein et al. (1957)
No OCA	Mean ± SD	18.0 ± 14.0 (50)	—	—	—	Rose et al. (1973)
+OCA	Mean ± SD	25.0 ± 21.0 (80)	—	—	—	Horwitt et al. (1975)
Cystathionine excretion (after 3-g L-methionine load) (μM/24 h)	Preload	18.3 ± 2.8 (6)	—	35.3 ± 6.2 (6)	—	Krishnaswamy (1972)
	Postload	44.6 ± 5.7 (6)	—	165.3 ± 13.0 (6)	—	Krishnaswamy (1972)
Erythrocyte pyridoxal phosphate (ng/million cells)	Average	0.32 ± 0.02 (60)	—	0.16 ± 0.01 (51)	—	Wachstein et al. (1957)
	Range	0.11–0.79		0.01–0.36		

[a]Values in parentheses indicate number of subjects studied.

137

establish whether a deficiency exists and, if so, whether the deficiency is due to an impaired absorption of the vitamin.

Procedures proposed for evaluating vitamin B_{12} status include serum and erythrocyte levels of vitamin B_{12}, urinary excretion of aminoimidazolecarboxamide (AIC), formiminoglutamic acid (FiGlu), or methylmalonic acid (MMA) and plasma disappearance rate of intravenously injected vitamin B_{12} (Sauberlich et al., 1974). Of these procedures, the determination of the serum vitamin B_{12} level has been the most useful and reliable. Microbiological assay methods or radioassay procedures are used for this purpose.

Since a close interrelationship exists between vitamin B_{12} and folacin, vitamin B_{12} nutritional status must be evaluated also in terms of folacin nutrition (Lowenstein et al., 1966; Kahn, 1970; Nixon and Bertino, 1970; Cook et al., 1971). In folacin deficiency, serum vitamin B_{12} levels may be low, but usually the levels are still above those found in patients with pernicious anemia. In these subjects, serum vitamin B_{12} levels return to normal following folate treatment. In contrast, in pernicious anemia, serum folate levels may be elevated, while erythrocyte folate levels may be low. Thus, both serum vitamin B_{12} and serum folate levels should be determined (Sauberlich et al., 1974). If a normal vitamin B_{12} level is found in the presence of a low serum folate level, a diagnosis of pernicious anemia is improbable. Low serum vitamin B_{12} levels in the absence of a folacin deficiency are indicative of pernicious anemia. The use of a Schilling test can determine whether the abnormal vitamin B_{12} status is the result of a lack of intrinsic factor, another form of malabsorption, or is a nutritional deficiency of vitamin B_{12}.

Serum vitamin B_{12} levels have been observed to fall markedly during pregnancy (Young et al., 1959; Ball and Giles, 1964; Metz et al., 1965; Baker et al., 1975). Metz et al. (1965) noted a fall in vitamin B_{12} levels of approximately 100 pg/ml of serum, although the mean serum vitamin B_{12} level was approximately 300 pg/ml at delivery. The levels rose to normal within 6 wk postpartum. Vitamin B_{12} supplementation did not change the pattern (Metz et al., 1965; Lowenstein et al., 1966; Cook et al., 1971). However, this fall did not occur during pregnancy in patients with initial subnormal serum vitamin B_{12} levels (Roberts et al., 1973). Morphological blood abnormalities were observed in many cases. Evidence suggests that the fall in serum vitamin B_{12} levels frequently observed in pregnancy represents in part a change in vitamin B_{12} metabolism independent of the dietary intake of vitamin B_{12} and does not necessarily reflect depletion of maternal vitamin B_{12} stores (Rothman, 1970). Changes in serum binders for vitamin B_{12} may be involved in the pathogenesis of the observed fall in serum levels of the vitamin during pregnancy (Green *et al.*, 1975). In some instances, inadequate folate nutrition may have depressed serum vitamin B_{12} levels (Rothman, 1970). Nevertheless, it cannot be discounted that the fall in serum vitamin B_{12} levels in pregnancy reflects, in part, depletion of maternal vitamin B_{12} stores. Edelstein and Metz (1969) observed a correlation between the serum vitamin B_{12} concentration and the level of the stores of the vitamin in muscle in late pregnancy. Erythrocyte vitamin B_{12} levels also tend to be subnormal in pregnant women (Harrison, 1972).

Laboratory indices for vitamin B_{12} nutritional status in the adult female are given in Table 6-9.

VITAMIN D

Vitamin D is required by humans of all ages, but the greatest need for the vitamin appears to exist in infants and children. Hence, vitamin D deficiency is very uncommon in the adult human unless exposure to sunlight is restricted (Wasserman and Corradino, 1973; DeLuca, 1974). Methods for assessing vitamin D status have been limited and unsatisfactory; consequently, knowledge concerning the metabolism of the vitamin during pregnancy has been largely conjectural.

The activity of serum alkaline phosphatase is increased in vitamin D deficiency. Serum alkaline phosphatase may increase somewhat during pregnancy, particularly during the third trimester, because of the production of a heat-stable placental alkaline phosphatase (Hodgkin *et al.*, 1973; Jones *et al.*, 1975; Morse *et al.*, 1975). Numerous procedures are available for measuring alkaline phosphatases in serum (Sauberlich *et al.*, 1974).

The principal circulating metabolite of vitamin D in human plasma is 25-hydroxycholecalciferol. Several competitive protein-binding assays are now available for measuring 25-hydroxycholecalciferol (Belsey *et al.*, 1971, 1974; Haddad and Chyu, 1971; Edelstein *et al.*, 1974; Haddad and Stamp, 1974; Rosen *et al.*, 1974). Assays for the more active metabolite 1,25-dihydroxycholecalciferol (Eisman *et al.*, 1976; Hughes *et al.*, 1976) also have been developed.

Serum levels of 25-hydroxylcholecalciferol in pregnant women have been reported to vary with ethnic and racial background (Dent and Gupta, 1975; Turton *et al.*, 1977), vegetarian dietary practice (Dent and Gupta, 1975), and season (Hillman and Haddad, 1976). However, pregnancy *per se* does not appear to cause any change in serum 25-hydroxycholecalciferol levels (Dent and Gupta, 1975). Vitamin D and its 25-hydroxy metabolite are transported in plasma by a specific

TABLE 6-9 Biochemical Assessment of Vitamin B_{12} Nutritional Status in the Adult Female

Test	Special Conditions	Display	Nonpregnant	Pregnancy Trimester			Post-partum	References
				1	2	3		
Serum vitamin B_{12} (pg/ml)		Mean ± SD	498 ± 95.7 (15)[a]	–	–	–	–	Hall et al. (1975)
		Mean ± SD	458 ± 200 (348)	–	–	–	–	Sauberlich (1976c)
		Range	100–1,350					
	Lactovegetarians	Mean ± SE	155 ± 26 (8)				–	Inamdar-Deshmukh et al. (1976)
	Nonvegetarians	Mean ± SE	331 ± 64 (11)				–	Inamdar-Deshmukh et al. (1976)
		Mean	214–1,150 (range)	420 (117)	360 (117)	310 (117)	475 (117)	Metz et al. (1965)
		Mean ± SD	–	–	–	–	236 ± 106 (30)	Pinto et al. (1973)
		Mean ± SD	–	224 ± 115 (320)	–	182 ± 96 (119)	–	Roberts et al. (1973)
		Range		44–696		36–468		
		Mean	–	267 (24)	260 (37)	190 (26)	433 (24)	Green et al. (1975)

140

					Reference
Chinese	Mean ± SD	—	—	267 ± 111 (326)	Hibbard and Hibbard (1972)
Malay	Mean ± SD	—	—	293 ± 109 (53)	Hibbard and Hibbard (1972)
Indian	Mean ± SD	—	—	219 ± 105 (26)	Green et al. (1975)
No OCA	Mean ± SD	690 ± 290 (72)	—	—	
+OCA	Mean ± SD	480 ± 240 (77)	—	—	
Erythrocyte vitamin B_{12} (pg/ml)					
Lactovegetarians	Mean ± SE	178 ± 68 (8)	—	—	Inamdar-Deshmukh et al. (1976)
Nonvegetarians	Mean ± SE	156 ± 19 (11)	—	—	Inamdar-Deshmukh et al. (1976)
	Mean ± SD	155 ± 35	133 ± 20 (13)	—	Harrison (1972)
	Range	100–220	104–180	—	

[a]Values in parentheses indicate number of subjects studied.

141

binding protein (Imawari *et al.*, 1976), and the binding capacity of maternal serum increases during pregnancy (Haddad *et al.*, 1976).

Laboratory indices for vitamin D nutritional status in the adult female are given in Table 6-10.

VITAMIN E

Erythrocyte hemolysis tests provide indirect information concerning vitamin E status, while more direct information can be obtained by measuring tocopherol levels in plasma or serum (Darby *et al.*, 1953b; Horwitt *et al.*, 1972; Leonard *et al.*, 1972; Sauberlich *et al.*, 1974). Serum tocopherol level may rise an average of 40–50 percent during pregnancy and return to normal prepregnancy levels postpartum (Darby *et al.*, 1953b; Ferguson *et al.*, 1955; Gordon *et al.*, 1958; Leonard *et al.*, 1972; Vobecky *et al.*, 1974a). This rise does not appear to occur until the second trimester of pregnancy (Ferguson *et al.*, 1955). Since these increases are observed without any changes in dietary intake of vitamin E, the observations appear to reflect a metabolic phenomena associated with changes in lipid transport during pregnancy (Darby *et al.*, 1953b; Horwitt *et al.*, 1972, 1975). Nevertheless, low dietary intakes of vitamin E are associated with lower plasma tocopherol levels (Ferguson *et al.*, 1955). As the plasma vitamin E level in the mothers is increased, an increase occurs in the vitamin E level in the plasma of the infants (Leonard *et al.*, 1972) and in the cord blood (Mino and Nishino, 1973). The use of oral contraceptive agents has been considered to give rise to increased plasma vitamin E levels as a probable consequence of increases in transport proteins (Horwitt *et al.*, 1975; Yeung and Chan, 1975). Various procedures have been described for performing the erythrocyte hemolysis test (Gyorgy *et al.*, 1952; Sauberlich *et al.*, 1974) and for measuring plasma tocopherol levels (Hansen and Warwick, 1969; Thompson *et al.*, 1973; Sauberlich *et al.*, 1974).

Laboratory indices for vitamin E nutritional status in the adult female are given in Table 6-11.

VITAMIN K

Although vitamin K is required by the adult human to maintain prothrombin and other factors necessary for normal blood clotting, a dietary deficiency of the vitamin uncomplicated by other factors is considered to be rare (Owen *et al.*, 1969; Quick, 1970; Rossi, 1972; Food and Nutrition Board, 1974; Sauberlich *et al.*, 1974). Such a

TABLE 6-10 Biochemical Assessment of Vitamin D Nutritional Status in the Adult Female

Test	Special Conditions	Display	Nonpregnant	Pregnancy Trimester			Post-partum	References
				1	2	3		
Total serum alkaline phosphatase								
Bodansky units/dl		Mean ± SE	—	1.95 ± 0.16 (61)[a]	2.58 ± 0.13 (97)	5.72 ± 0.14 (80)	3.28 ± 0.14 (95)	Morse et al. (1975)
Bodansky units/dl		Mean ± SE	3.71 ± 0.58 (21)	3.81 ± 1.64 (17)	4.72 ± 1.81 (67)	8.18 ± 3.25 (102)	—	Iyengar and Srikantia (1970)
King-Armstrong units/dl	Asian female	Mean ± SD	8.5 ± 3.4 (27)	—	8.2 ± 3.3 (16)	16.8 ± 5.1 (22)-	—	Hodgkin et al. (1973)
	Caucasian female		7.7 ± 2.9 (23)					
	Caucasians	Mean ± SD	6.4 ± 0.6 (20)	6.4 ± 1.3 (14)	7.5 ± 1.3 (14)	13.4 ± 1.9 (14)	—	Dent and Gupta (1975)
	Asians Vegetarian	Mean ± SD	6.7 ± 1.8 (18)	6.4 ± 1.1 (23)	9.5 ± 1.7 (23)	16.0 ± 1.8 (23)	—	Dent and Gupta (1975)
	Non vegetarian	Mean ± SD	6.2 ± 1.0 (16)	6.2 ± 0.9 (16)	9.8 ± 1.8 (16)	15.0 ± 1.7 (16)	—	Dent and Gupta (1975)

TABLE 6-10 (Continued)

Test	Special Conditions	Display	Nonpregnant	Pregnancy Trimester			Post-partum	References
				1	2	3		
Serum 25-hy-droxycholecal-ciferol (ng/ml)		Mean ± SE	—	—	22.3 ± 1.5 (3)	24.4 ± 8.0 (7)	—	Hillman and Haddad (1974)
	Caucasians	Mean ± SE	—	—	—	31.0 ± 11.5 (14)	—	Hillman and Haddad (1974)
	Blacks	Mean ± SE	—	—	—	22.1 ± 9.7 (20)	—	Hillman and Haddad (1974)
	Adults—male & female	Mean ± SD	18.8 ± 7.6 (81)	—	—	—	—	Haddad and Stamp (1974)
		Mean ± SE	—	—	—	28.0 ± 2.0 (15)	—	Rosen et al. (1974)
	Adults—male & female	Mean ± SD	15.2 ± 5.6 (18)	—	—	—	—	Edelstein et al. (1974)
	Normal subjects	Mean ± SE	35.2 ± 3.6 (15)	—	—	—	—	Belsey et al. (1971, 1974)
		Range	20–100					

144

Caucasians	Mean ± SD	13.9 ± 2.0 (20)	20.4 ± 4.8 (14)	16.7 ± 3.0 (14)	15.0 ± 2.2 (14)	—	Dent and Gupta (1975)
Asians Vegetarian	Mean ± SD	6.7 ± 1.8 (18)	9.0 ± 3.2 (23)	9.2 ± 2.4 (23)	7.4 ± 1.7 (23)	—	Dent and Gupta (1975)
Nonvegetarian	Mean ± SD	11.3 ± 1.8 (16)	10.7 ± 2.2 (16)	10.1 ± 16 (16)	9.8 ± 1.2 (16)	—	Dent and Gupta (1975)
Israelis Negev Bedouins	Mean ± SD	25.4 ± 9.78 (12)	—	—	23.4 ± 8.52 (19)	—	Shany et al. (1976)
Bersheeba	Mean ± SD	32.7 ± 6.02 (7)	—	—	44.3 ± 9.24 (12)	—	Shany et al. (1976)
Plasma α-1, 25-dihydroxy-cholecalciferol (ng/dl)							
Normal adults; male & female	Mean ± SD	3.3 ± 0.6 (78)	—	—	—	—	Hughes et al. (1976)
Normal adults	Range Mean ± SE	2.1–4.5 2.9 ± 0.2 (5)	—	—	—	—	Eisman et al. (1976)

^{a}Values in parentheses indicate number of subjects studied.

TABLE 6-11 Biochemical Assessment of Vitamin E Nutritional Status in the Adult Female

| Test | Special Conditions | Display | Nonpregnant | Pregnancy Trimester | | | Post-partum | References |
				1	2	3		
Serum α-tocopherol (mg/dl)		Mean ± SD	0.89 ± 0.20 (74)[a]	1.04 ± 0.23 (240)	1.16 ± 0.24 (273)	1.32 ± 0.29 (149)	0.93 ± 0.28 (35)	Darby et al. (1953b); Ferguson et al. (1955)
		Mean ± SD	1.23 ± 0.27 (74)	–	–	–	–	Wei Wo and Draper (1975)
		Mean ± SD	–	0.62 ± 0.26 (108)	0.77 ± 0.27 (250)	0.96 ± 0.29 (503)	–	Vobecky et al. (1974a)
		Mean ± SE	–	–	–	1.71 ± 0.17 (57)	–	Mino and Nishino (1973)
		Mean ± SD	–	–	–	0.92 ± 0.29 (200)	–	Leonard et al. (1972)
			0.84	–	–	–	1.32 (20)	Gordon et al. (1958)
	No OCA	Mean ± SE	0.96 ± 0.04 (32)	–	–	1.36 ± 0.06 (22)	0.88 ± 0.10 (11)	Horwitt et al. (1975)
	+OCA	Mean ± SE	0.98 ± 0.05 (15)	–	–	–	–	
Erythrocyte H₂O₂ hemolysis (%)		Mean ± SD	13 ± 22 (315)	–	–	–	–	Sauberlich (1976a)
		Range	0–99					

[a] Values in parentheses indicate number of subjects studied.

146

TABLE 6-12 Biochemical Assessment of Pantothenic Acid Nutritional Status in the Adult Female

Test	Display	Nonpregnant	Pregnancy trimester			Post-partum	References
			1	2	3		
Whole-blood total pantothenate (μg/dl)	Mean ± SD	183 ± 60 (4)[a]	–	–	103 ± 26 (17)	112 ± 26 (13)	Cohenour and Calloway (1972)
	Range	105–242			60–145	85–172	
Free blood pantothenate (μg/dl blood)	Mean	9.7 (39)	–	–	–	–	Ishiguro (1972)
Bound blood pantothenate (μg/dl blood)	Mean	96.4 (39)	–	–	–	–	Ishiguro (1972)
Urinary free pantothenate mg/g creatinine	Mean ± SD	2.3 ± 0.7 (5)	–	–	–	3.8 ± 1.8 (14)	Cohenour and Calloway (1972)
	Range	1.6–3.3				1.4–6.7	
mg/24 h	Mean ± SD	2.5 ± 0.8 (5)	–	–	–	3.5 ± 1.6 (14)	Cohenour and Calloway (1972)
	Range	1.4–3.5				1.0–5.2	

[a]Values in parentheses indicate number of subjects studied.

147

deficiency most commonly occurs in situations in which there is malabsorption of fat-soluble materials or if prolonged antibiotic therapy has altered the gut bacterial flora. A prolonged prothrombin time results because of decreased activities of factor VII and prothrombin. Factor IX level is also decreased, and a prolonged partial thromboplastin time occurs. In order to distinguish vitamin K deficiency from the causes of prolonged prothrombin and partial thromboplastin times, specific factor assays may be done. The simplest confirmation of vitamin K deficiency is the rapid return of an abnormal prothrombin time to normal when vitamin K is given parenterally.

PANTOTHENIC ACID

Information is limited on the biochemical assessment of pantothenic acid status in pregnancy (Ishiguro, 1962; Cohenour and Calloway, 1972; Markkanen, 1973; Sauberlich et al., 1974). Pantothenic acid levels in blood appear to fall during pregnancy and slowly return to normal postpartum (Ishiguro, 1962, 1972; Cohenour and Calloway, 1972). Since most of the pantothenic acid in blood is present in the erythrocyte, any changes in hematocrit must be considered in evaluating pantothenic acid status based on whole-blood levels. Until additional information and techniques become available, the indices presented here must be considered tentative at best.

Laboratory indices for pantothenic acid nutritional status in the adult female are given in Table 6-12.

REFERENCES

Adams, P. W., J. Folkard, V. Wynn, and M. Seed. 1976. Influence of oral contraceptives, pyridoxine (vitamin B_6), and tryptophan on carbohydrate metabolism. Lancet 1:759–764.

Avery, B., and W. J. Ledger. 1970. Folic acid metabolism in well-nourished pregnant women. Obstet. Gynecol. 35:616–624.

Baker, H., and O. Frank. 1968. Vitamin B_6, p. 66. In Clinical Vitaminology. Interscience Publishers, New York. p. 66.

Baker, H., O. Frank, A. D. Thomson, A. Langer, E. D. Munves, B. DeAngelis, and H. A. Kaminetzky. 1975. Vitamin profiles of 174 mothers and newborns at parturition. Am. J. Clin. Nutr. 28:56–65.

Ball, E. W., and C. Giles. 1964. Folic acid and vitamin B_{12} levels in pregnancy and their relation to megaloblastic anemia. J. Clin. Pathol. 17:165–174.

Balmelli, G. P., and H-J. Huser. 1974. Zur frage des Folsauremangels bei Schwangeren in der Schweiz. Schweiz. Med. Wochenschr. 104:351–356.

Bamji, M. S. 1970. Transketolase activity and urinary excretion of thiamin in the assessment of thiamin-nutrition status of Indians. Am. J. Clin. Nutr. 23:52–58.

Bamji, M. S. 1976. Enzymic evaluation of thiamin, riboflavin and pyridoxine status of parturient women and their newborn infants. Br. J. Nutr. 35:259–265.

Basu, S. R. J., and R. Arulanantham. 1973. A study of serum protein and retinol levels in pregnancy and toxaemia of pregnancy in women of low socio-economic status. Indian J. Med. Res. 61:589–595.

Bayoumi, R. A., and S. B. Rosalki. 1976. Evaluation of methods of coenzyme activation of erythrocyte enzymes for detection of deficiency of vitamins B_1, B_2, and B_6. Clin. Chem. 22:327–335.

Belsey, R., H. F. DeLuca, and J. T. Potts. 1971. Competitive binding assay for vitamin D and 25-OH vitamin D. J. Clin. Endocrinol. Metab. 33:554–557.

Belsey, R. E., H. F. DeLuca, and J. T. Potts, Jr. 1974. A rapid assay for 25-OH-vitamin D_3 without preparative chromatography. J. Clin. Endocrinol. Metab. 38:1046–1051.

Blakley, R. L. 1969. The Biochemistry of Folic Acid and Related Pteridines. Vol. 13, Frontiers of Biology. A. Neuberger and E. L. Tatum, ed. North-Holland Publishing Co., Amsterdam (Wiley Interscience, New York, distributors). 570 pp.

Brin, M. 1971. Abnormal tryptophan metabolism in pregnancy and with oral contraceptive pill. II. Relative levels of vitamin B_6-vitamers in cord and maternal blood. Am. J. Clin. Nutr. 24:704–708.

Brin, M. C., M. V. Dibble, A. Peel, E. McMullen, A. Bourquin, and N. Chen. 1965. Some preliminary findings on the nutritional status of the aged in Onondaga County, New York. Am. J. Clin. Nutr. 17:240–258.

Brook, M., and J. J. Grimshaw. 1968. Vitamin C concentration of plasma and leukocytes as related to smoking habit, age, and sex of humans. Am. J. Clin. Nutr. 21:1254–1258.

Brophy, M. H., and P. K. Siiteri. 1976. Pyridoxal phosphate and hypertensive disorders of pregnancy. Am. J. Obstet. Gynecol. 121:1075–1079.

Brown, R. R. 1972. Normal and pathological conditions which may alter the human requirements for vitamin B_6 nutriture of her newborn infant. Z. Kinderheilk. 115:163–164.

Brown, R. R., M. J. Thornton, and J. M. Price. 1961. The effect of vitamin supplementation on the urinary excretion of tryptophan metabolites by pregnant women. J. Clin. Invest. 40:617–623.

Brown, R. R., D. P. Rose, J. E. Leklem, H. Linkswiler, and R. Anand. 1975. Urinary 4-pyridoxic acid, plasma pyridoxal phosphate, and erythrocyte aminotransferase levels in oral conceptive users receiving controlled intakes of vitamin B_6. Am. J. Clin. Nutr. 28:10–19.

Canham, J. E., E. M. Baker, N. Raica, Jr., and H. E. Sauberlich. 1966. Vitamin B_6 requirement of adult men. Proc. VII Int. Congr. Nutr. Hamburg, 5:558–562. Pergamon Press, Elmsford, N.Y.

Chabner, B., and D. Livingston. 1970. A simple enzymic assay for pyridoxal phosphate. Anal. Biochem. 34:413–423.

Chanarin, I., D. Rothman, A. Ward, and J. Perry. 1968. Folate status and requirement in pregnancy. Br. Med. J. 2:390–394.

Cheney, M., Z. I. Sabry, and G. H. Beaton. 1965. Erythrocyte glutanic-pyruvic transaminase activity in man. Am. J. Clin. Nutr. 16:337–338.

Chong, Y. H., and G. S. Ho. 1970. Erythrocyte transketolase activity. Am. J. Clin. Nutr. 23:261–266.

Cleary, R. E., L. Lumeng, and T-K. Li. 1975. Maternal and fetal plasma levels of pyridoxal phosphate at term: adequacy of vitamin B_6 supplementation during pregnancy. Am. J. Obstet. Gynecol. 121:25–28.

Cohenour, S. H., and D. H. Calloway. 1972. Blood, urine, and dietary pantothenic acid levels of pregnant teenagers. Am. J. Clin. Nutr. 25:512–517.

Colman, N., M. Barker, R. Green, and J. Metz. 1974. Prevention of folate deficiency in pregnancy by fortification. Am. J. Clin. Nutr. 27:339–344.

Colman, N., J. V. Larsen, M. Barker, E. A. Barker, R. Green, and J. Metz. 1975. Prevention of folate deficiency by food fortification. III. Effect in pregnant subjects of varying amounts of added folic acid. Am. J. Clin. Nutr. 28:465–470.

Contractor, S. F., and B. Shane. 1970. Blood and urine levels of vitamin B_6 in the mother and fetus before and after loading of the mother with vitamin B_6. Am. J. Obstet. Gynecol. 107:635–640.

Cook, J. D., J. Alvarado, A. Gutniskey et al. 1971. Nutritional deficiency and anemia in Latin America: a collaborative study. Blood 38:591–603.

Cooperman, J. M., H. S. Cole, M. Gordon, and R. Lopez. 1973. Erythrocyte glutathione reductase as a measure of riboflavin nutritional status of pregnant women and newborns. Proc. Soc. Exp. Biol. Med. 143:326–328.

Darby, W. J., R. O. Cannon, and M. M. Kaser. 1948. The biochemical assessment of nutritional status during pregnancy. Obstet. Gynecol. Survey 3:704.

Darby, W. J., P. M. Densen, R. O. Cannon et al. 1953a. The Vanderbilt cooperative study of maternal and infant nutrition. I. Background. II. Methods. III. Description of the sample and data. J. Nutr. 51:539–563.

Darby, W. J., W. J. McGanity, M. P. Martin et al. 1953b. The Vanderbilt cooperative study of maternal and infant nutrition. IV. Dietary, laboratory and physical findings in 2,129 delivered pregnancies. J. Nutr. 51:565–597.

De Lange, D. J., and C. P. Joubert. 1964. Assessment of nicotinic acid status of population groups. Am. J. Clin. Nutr. 15:169–174.

DeLuca, H. F. 1974. Vitamin D: the vitamin and the hormone. Fed. Proc. 33:2211–2219.

Dent, C. E., and M. M. Gupta. 1975. Plasma 25-hydroxyvitamin-D levels during pregnancy in Caucasians and in vegetarian and nonvegetarian Asians. Lancet II:1057–1060.

Edelstein, T., and J. Metz. 1969. Correlation between vitamin B_{12} concentration in serum and muscle in late pregnancy. J. Obstet. Gynaecol. Br. Commonw. 76:545–548.

Edelstein, S., M. Charman, D. E. M. Lawson, and E. Kodicek. 1974. Competitive protein-binding assay for 25-hydroxycholecalciferol. Clin. Sci. Mol. Med. 46:231–240.

Edozien, J. C., B. R. Switzer, and R. B. Bryan. 1976. Medical evaluation of the special supplemental food program for women, infants and children. Vol. II. Results. Department of Nutrition, School of Public Health, University of North Carolina, Chapel Hill, N.C., July 15, 1976. pp. 409, 411.

Eichner, E. R., C. J. Paine, V. L. Dickson, and M. D. Hargrove, Jr. 1975. Clinical and laboratory observations on serum folate-binding protein. Blood 46:599–609.

Eisman, J. A., A. J. Hamstra, B. E. Kream, and H. F. DeLuca. 1976. 1-25-Dihydroxyvitamin D in biological fluids: a simplified and sensitive assay. Science 193:1021–1023.

Ferguson, M. E., E. Bridgeforth, M. L. Duaife, M. P. Martin, R. O. Cannon, W. J. McGanity, J. Newbill, and W. J. Darby. 1955. The Vanderbilt cooperative study of maternal and infant nutrition. VII. Tocopherol in relation to pregnancy. J. Nutr. 55:305–321.

Fleming, A. F. 1972. Urinary excretion of folate in pregnancy. J. Obstet. Gynaecol. Br. Commonw. 79:916–920.

Food and Nutrition Board (National Research Council). 1974. Recommended dietary allowances, 8th ed. National Academy of Sciences, Washington, D.C. 129 pp.

Gajwani, B. W., B. C. Patel, A. S. Mehta, R. V. Bhatt, R. S. Pande, and K. Venugopal. 1969. Anemias of pregnancy. J. Indian Med. Assoc. 52:420–423.

Gal, I., and C. E. Parkinson. 1972. Variations in the pattern of maternal serum vitamin A and carotenoids during human reproduction. Int. J. Vit. Nutr. Res. 42:565–575.

Gal, I., and C. E. Parkinson. 1974. Effects of nutrition and other factors on pregnant women's serum vitamin A levels. Am. J. Clin. Nutr. 27:688–695.

Garcia, P. A., W. D. Brewer, C. W. Merritt, and H. B. Mead. 1974. Nutritional status of adolescent primigravidae. II. Blood indices during pregnancy and postpartum. Iowa State J. Res. 48:219–229.

Glover, J. 1973. Retinol-binding proteins. Vit. Horm. 31:1–42.

Gordon, H. H., H. M. Nitowsky, J. T. Tildon, and S. Levin. 1958. Studies of tocopherol deficiency in infants and children. V. An interim study. Pediatrics 21:673–681.

Green, R., N. Colman, and J. Metz. 1975. Comparison of results of microbiologic and radioisotopic assays for serum vitamin B_{12} during pregnancy. Am. J. Obstet. Gynecol. 122:21–24.

Gyorgy, P., G. Cogan, and C. S. Rose. 1952. Availability of vitamin E in the newborn infant. Proc. Soc. Exp. Biol. Med. 81:536–538.

Haddad, J., and K. J. Chyu. 1971. Competitive protein binding radioassay for 25-hydroxycholecalciferol. J. Clin. Endocrinol. 33:992.

Haddad, J. G., and C. B. Stamp. 1974. Circulating 25-hydroxyvitamin D in man. Am. J. Med. 57:57–62.

Haddad, J. G., L. Hillman, and S. Zojanasathit. 1976. Human serum binding capacity and affinity for 25-hydroxyergocalciferol and 25-hydroxycholecalciferol. J. Clin. Endocrinol. Metab. 43:86–91.

Hall, C. A., S. A. Bardwell, E. S. Allen, and M. E. Rappozzo. 1975. Variation in plasma folate levels among groups of healthy persons. Am. J. Clin. Nutr. 28:854–857.

Hamfelt, A., and L. Hahn. 1969. Pyridoxal phosphate concentration in plasma and tryptophan load test during pregnancy. Clin. Chim. Acta 25:91–96.

Hamfelt, A., and T. Tuvemo. 1972. Pyridoxal phosphate and folic acid concentration in blood and erythrocyte aspartate amino-transferase activity during pregnancy. Clin. Chim. Acta 41:287–298.

Hansen, L. G., and W. J. Warwick. 1969. A fluorometric micromethod for serum vitamins A and E. Am. J. Clin. Pathol. 51:538–541.

Harrison, R. J. 1972. Erythrocyte vitamin B_{12} levels in pregnancy. J. Obstet. Gynaecol. Br. Commonw. 79:226–227.

Health Services and Mental Health Administration. 1972. Ten-State Nutrition Study, 1968–1970. IV. Biochemical. U.S. Department of Health, Education, and Welfare, Center for Disease Control, Atlanta, Ga. DHEW Publication No. (HSM) 72-8132, pp. IV-146, IV-202, IV-221, IV-253.

Heller, S., R. M. Salkeld, and W. F. Korner. 1973. Vitamin B_6 status in pregnancy. Am. J. Clin. Nutr. 26:1339–1348.

Heller, S., R. M. Salkeld, and W. F. Korner. 1974. Vitamin B_1 status in pregnancy. Am. J. Clin. Nutr. 27:1221–1224.

Henshaw, J. L., G. Noakes, S. O. Morris, M. Bennion, and C. J. Gubler. 1970. Method for evaluating thiamine adequacy in college women. J. Am. Diet. Assoc. 57:436–441.

Herbert, V. 1965. Folic acid. Annu. Rev. Med. 16:359–370.

Hershko, C., N. Grossowicz, M. Rachmilewitz, S. Kesten, and G. Izak. 1975. Serum and erythrocyte folates in combined iron and folate deficiency. Am. J. Clin. Nutr. 28:1217–1222.

Hibbard, B. M., and E. D. Hibbard. 1972. Anaemia and folate status in late pregnancy in a mixed Asiatic population. J. Obstet. Gynaecol. Br. Commonw. 79:584–591.

Hillman, L. S., and J. G. Haddad. 1974. Human perinatal vitamin D metabolism. I. 25-Hydroxyvitamin D in maternal and cord blood. J. Pediatr. 84:742–749.

Hillman, L. S., and J. G. Haddad. 1976. Perinatal vitamin D metabolism. III. Factors influencing late gestational human serum 25-hydroxyvitamin D. Am. J. Obstet. Gynecol. 125:196–200.

Hodgkin, P., G. H. Kay, P. M. Hine, G. A. Lumb, and S. W. Stanbury. 1973. Vitamin D deficiency in Asians at home and in Britain. Lancet II:167–172.

Hoffbrand, A. V., B. F. A. Newcombe, and D. L. Mollin. 1966. Method of assay of red cell folate activity and the value of the assay as a test for folate deficiency. J. Clin. Pathol. 19:17–28.

Horwitt, M. K., C. C. Harvey, C. H. Dahm, Jr., and M. T. Searcy. 1972. Relationship between tocopherol and serum lipid levels for determination of nutritional adequacy. Ann. N.Y. Acad. Sci. 203:223–236.

Horwitt, M. K., C. C. Harvey, and C. H. Dahm, Jr. 1975. Relationship between levels of blood lipids, vitamins C, A, and E, serum copper compounds, and urinary excretions of tryptophan metabolites in women taking oral contraceptive therapy. Am. J. Clin. Nutr. 28:403–412.

Hughes, M. R., D. J. Baylink, P. G. Jones, and M. R. Haussler. 1976. Radioligand receptor assay for 25-hydroxyvitamin D_2/D_3 and 1α,25-dihydroxyvitamin D_2/D_3. J. Clin. Invest. 58:61–70.

Imawari, M., K. Kida, and D. S. Goodman. 1976. The transport of vitamin D and its 25-hydroxy metabolite in human plasma. Isolation and partial characterization of vitamin D and 25-hydroxyvitamin D binding protein. J. Clin. Invest. 58:514–523.

Inamdar-Deshmukh, A. B., V. S. Jathar, D. A. Joseph, and R. S. Satoskar. 1976. Erythrocyte vitamin B_{12} activity in healthy Indian lactovegetarians. Br. J. Haematol. 32:395–401.

Ishiguro, K. 1962. Blood pantothenic acid content of pregnant women. Tohoku J. Exp. Med. 78:7–10.

Ishiguro, K. 1972. Aging effect of blood pantothenic acid content in female. Tohoku J. Exp. Med. 107:367–372.

Iyengar, L. 1971. Folic acid requirements of Indian pregnant women. Am. J. Obstet. Gynecol. 111:13–16.

Iyengar, L. 1973. Oral lesions in pregnancy. Lancet I:680–681.

Iyengar, L., and S. G. Srikantia. 1970. Serum alkaline phosphatase in pregnancy. Am. J. Clin. Nutr. 23:68–72.

Jones, D. D., G. J. Williams, and B. Prochazka. 1975. The serum activity of glucose-6-phosphatase and 5′-nucleotidase during human pregnancy. Enzyme 19:233–243.

Joubert, C. P., and D. J. de Lange. 1962. A modification of the method for the determination of N′-methyl-2-pyridone-5-carboxylamide in human urine and its application in the evaluation of nicotinic acid status. Proc. Nutrition Soc. South. Afr. 3:60–65.

Kahn, S. B. 1970. Recent advances in the nutritional anemias. Med. Clin. North Am. 54:631–645.

Kitay, D. Z. 1969. Folic acid deficiency in pregnancy. Am. J. Obstet. Gynecol. 104:1067–1107.

Krishnaswamy, K. 1972. Methionine load test in pyridoxine deficiency. Int. J. Vit. Nutr. Res. 42:468–475.

Landon, M. J., and F. E. Hytten. 1971. The excretion of folate in pregnancy. J. Obstet. Gynaecol. Br. Commonw. 78:769–775.

Landon, M. J., and A. Oxley. 1971. Relation between maternal and infant blood folate activities. Arch. Dis. Child. 46:810–814.

Leklem, J. E. 1971. Quantitative aspects of tryptophan metabolism in human and other species: a review. Am. J. Clin. Nutr. 24:659–672.

Leonard, P. J., E. Doyle, and W. Harrington. 1972. Levels of vitamin E in the plasma of newborn infants and of the mothers. Am. J. Clin. Nutr. 25:480–484.

Lewis, J. M., O. Bodansky, M. C. C. Lillienfeld, and H. Schneider. 1974. Supplements of vitamin A and of carotene during pregnancy. Their effect on the levels of vitamin A and carotene in the blood of mother and of newborn infant. Am. J. Dis. Child. 73:143.

Linkswiler, H. 1967. Biochemical and physiological changes in vitamin B_6 deficiency. Am. J. Clin. Nutr. 20:547–557.

Lowenstein, L., L. Brunton, and Y-S. Hsieh. 1966. Nutritional anemia and megaloblastosis in pregnancy. Can. Med. Assoc. J. 94:636–645.

Luhby, A. L., M. Brin, M. Gordon, P. Davis, M. Murphy, and H. Spiegel. 1971. Vitamin B_6 metabolism in users of oral contraceptive agents. I. Abnormal urinary xanthurenic acid excretion and its correction by pyridoxine. Am. J. Clin. Nutr. 24:684–693.

Lumeng, L., R. E. Cleary, and T-K. Li. 1974. Effect of oral contraceptives on the plasma concentration of pyridoxal phosphate. Am. J. Clin. Nutr. 27:326–333.

Markkanen, T. 1973. The metabolic significance of pantothenic acid as assessed by its levels in serum in various clinical and experimental conditions. Int. J. Vit. Nutr. Res. 43:302–317.

Markkanen, T., R.-L. Pajula, P. Himanen, and S. Virtanen. 1973. Serum folic acid activity (*L. casei*) in Sephodex gel chromatography. J. Clin. Pathol. 26:486–493.

Massod, M. F., S. L. McGuire, and K. R. Werner. 1971. Analysis of blood transketolase activity. Am. J. Clin. Pathol. 55:465-470.

McGanity, W. J., H. M. Little, A. Fogelman, L. Jennings, E. Calhoun, and E. B. Dawson. 1969. Pregnancy in the adolescent. I. Preliminary summary of health status. Am. J. Obstet. Gynecol. 103:773–788.

McLeroy, V. J., and H. E. Schendel. 1973. Influence of oral contraceptives on ascorbic acid concentrations in healthy, sexually mature women. Am. J. Clin. Nutr. 26:191–196.

Metz, J., H. Festenstein, and P. Welch. 1965. Effect of folic acid and vitamin B_{12} supplementation on tests of folate and vitamin B_{12} nutrition in pregnancy. Am. J. Clin. Nutr. 16:472–479.

Migasena, P., S. Changbumrung, V. Supawan, and J. Limtrakarn. 1974. Erythrocyte transketolase activity in blood of mothers, umbilical cord and newborn babies in Thailand. J. Nutr. Sci. Vitaminol. 20:371–374.

Mino, M., and H. Nishino. 1973. Fetal and maternal relationship in serum vitamin E level. J. Nutr. Sci. Vitaminol. 19:475–482.

Morse, E. H., R. P. Clarke, D. E. Keyser, S. B. Merrow, and D. E. Bee. 1975. Comparison of the nutritional status of pregnant adolescents with adult pregnant women. I. Biochemical findings. Am. J. Clin. Nutr. 28:1000–1013.

al-Nagdy, S. A., A. K. Khattab, H. I. El Asghal, and K. Abdel Hady. 1971. Maternal and neonatal serum vitamin A levels in normal Egyptian subjects. Environmental Child Health, December, pp. 168–170.

Nichoalds, G. E., J. D. Lawrence, and H. E. Sauberlich. 1974. Assessment of status of riboflavin nutriture by assay of erythrocyte glutathione reductase activity. Clin. Chem. 20:624–628.

Nixon, P. F., and J. R. Bertino. 1970. Interrelationships of vitamin B_{12} and folate in man. Am. J. Med. 48:555–561.

Nutrition Survey of the Lower Greasewood Chapter Navajo Tribe, 1968–1969. Department of Community Medicine, University of Pittsburg and USPHS, Indian Health Service. 83 pp.

Owen, C. A., Jr., E. J. W. Bowie, P. Didisheim, and J. H. Thompson, Jr. 1969. The diagnosis of bleeding disorders. Little, Brown and Co., Boston, Mass. 300 pp.

Pinto, A. V., F. Santos, M. C. Midlej, A. M. Almeida, and M. P. Gama. 1973. Vitamin B_{12} and folic acid in maternal and newborn sera. Rev. Invest. Clin. 25:341–344.

Pritchard, J. A., D. E. Scott, and P. J. Whalley. 1971. Maternal folate deficiency and pregnancy wastage. IV. Effects of folic acid supplements, anticonvulsants, and oral contraceptives. Am. J. Obstet. Gynecol. 109:341–346.

Pulliam, R. P., W. N. Dannenburg, R. L. Burt, and N. H. Leake. 1962. Carotene and vitamin A in pregnancy and the early puerperium. Proc. Soc. Exp. Biol. Med. 109:913–916.

Quick, A. J. 1970. Bleeding problems in clinical medicine. W. B. Saunders Co., Philadelphia, Pa. 225 pp.

Raica, N., Jr., and H. E. Sauberlich. 1965. Blood cell transaminase activity in human vitamin B_6 deficiency. Am. J. Clin. Nutr. 15:67–72.

Reinken, L., H. Berger, O. Dapunt, and W. F. Korner. 1973. Relations between vitamin B_6 status of mother and vitamin B_6 nutriture of her newborn infant. Z. Kinderheilkd. 115:163–174.

Rivers, J. M. 1975. Oral contraceptives and ascorbic acid. Am. J. Clin. Nutr. 28:550–554.

Roberts, P. D., H. James, A. Petrie, J. O. Morgan, and A. V. Hoffrand. 1973. Vitamin B_{12} status in pregnancy among immigrants to Britain. Br. Med. J. 3:67–72.

Rodriguez, M. S., and M. I. Irwin. 1972. A conspectus of research on vitamin A requirements of man. J. Nutr. 102:909–968.

Rose, D. P., and I. P. Braidman. 1971. Excretion of tryptophan metabolites as affected by pregnancy, contraceptive steroids, and steroid hormones. Am. J. Clin. Nutr. 24:673–683.

Rose, D. P., R. Strong, J. Folkard, and P. W. Adams. 1973. Erythrocyte aminotransferase activities in women using oral contraceptives and the effect of vitamin B_6 supplementation. Am. J. Clin. Nutr. 26:48–52.

Rose, D. P., J. E. Leklem, R. R. Brown, and H. M. Linkswiler. 1975. Effect of oral contraceptives and vitamin B_6 deficiency on carbohydrate metabolism. Am. J. Clin. Nutr. 28:872–878.

Rosen, J. F., M. Roginsky, G. Nathenson, and L. Finberg. 1974. 25-Hydroxyvitamin D: plasma levels in mothers and their premature infants with neonatal hypocalcemia. Am. J. Dis. Child. 127:220–223.

Rosenthal, H. L., G. A. Goldsmith, and H. P. Sarett. 1953. Excretion on N^1-methylnicotinamide and the 6-pyridone of N^1-methylnicotinamide in urine of human subjects. Proc. Soc. Exp. Biol. Med. 84:208–211.

Rossi, E. C. (guest editor). 1972. Symposium on hemorrhagic disorders. Med. Clin. North Am. 56(1):1–289.

Rothman, D. 1970. Folic acid in pregnancy. Am. J. Obstet. Gynecol. 108:149–175.

Sauberlich, H. E. 1967. Biochemical alternations in thiamine deficiency—their interpretation. Am. J. Clin. Nutr. 20:528–542.

Sauberlich, H. E. 1975. Vitamin C status: methods and findings. Ann. N.Y. Acad. Sci. 258:438–450.

Sauberlich, H. E. 1976a. Unpublished data.

Sauberlich, H. E. 1976b. Unpublished data from Ten-State Nutrition Survey.

Sauberlich, H. E. 1976c. Detection of folic acid deficiency in populations, pp. 213–231. In H. P. Broquist, C. E. Butterworth, Jr., and C. Wagner, ed., Folic Acid: Biochemistry and Physiology in Relation to the Human Nutrition Requirement. National Academy of Sciences, Washington, D.C.

Sauberlich, H. E., and J. E. Canham. 1973. Vitamin B_6. In R. S. Goodhart and M. E. Shils, ed., Modern Nutrition in Health and Disease, 5th ed. Lea and Febiger, Philadelphia.

Sauberlich, H. E., J. E. Canham, E. M. Baker, N. Raica, Jr., and Y. F. Herman. 1970. Human vitamin B_6 nutriture. J. Sci. Ind. Res. 29:S28–S37.

Sauberlich, H. E., J. E. Canham, E. M. Baker, N. Raica, Jr., and Y. F. Herman. 1972. Biochemical assessment of the nutritional status of vitamin B₆ in the human. Am. J. Clin. Nutr. 25:629–642.

Sauberlich, H. E., R. P. Dowdy, and J. H. Skala. 1974. Laboratory tests for the assessment of nutritional status. CRC Press, Cleveland, Ohio. 136 pp.

Sauberlich, H. E., W. C. Goad, J. H. Skala, and P. P. Waring. 1976. Procedure for mechanized (continuous-flow) measurement of serum ascorbic acid (vitamin C). Clin. Chem. 22:105–110.

Shane, B., and S. F. Contractor. 1975. Assessment of vitamin B₆ status. Studies on pregnant women and oral contraceptive users. Am. J. Clin. Nutr. 28:739–747.

Shany, S., J. Hirsh, and G. M. Berlyne. 1976. 25-Hydroxycholecalciferol levels in Bedouins in the Negev. Am. J. Clin. Nutr. 29:1104–1107.

Shojania, A. M., and G. J. Hornady. 1973. Oral contraceptives and folate absorption. J. Lab. Clin. Med. 82:869–875.

Smeets, E. H. J., H. Muller, and J. DeWael. 1971. A NADH-dependent transketolase assay in erythrocyte hemolysates. Clin. Chim. Acta 33:379–386.

Smith, F. R., D. S. Goodman, G. Grroyave, and F. Viteri. 1973. Serum vitamin A, retinol-binding protein, and prealbumin concentration in protein-calorie malnutrition. II. Treatment including supplemental vitamin A. Am. J. Clin. Nutr. 26:982–987.

Smith, J. L., G. A. Goldsmith, and J. D. Lawrence. 1975. Effects of oral contraceptive steroids on vitamin and lipid levels in serum. Am. J. Clin. Nutr. 28:371–376.

Solomon, E., S. L. Lee, M. Wasserman, and J. Malkin. 1962. Association of anaemia in pregnancy and folic acid deficiency. J. Obstet. Gynaecol. Br. Commonw. 69:724–728.

Sprince, H., R. S. Lowy, C. E. Folsome, and E. J. Behrman. 1951. Studies on the urinary excretion of "xanthurenic acid" during normal and abnormal pregnancy: a survey of the excretion of "xanthurenic acid" in normal nonpregnant, normal pregnant, pre-eclamptic, and eclamptic women. Am. J. Obstet. Gynecol. 62:84–92.

Stone, M. L., A. L. Luhby, R. Feldman, M. Gordon, and J. M. Cooperman. 1967. Folic acid metabolism in pregnancy. Am. J. Obstet. Gynecol. 99:638–648.

Suthutvoravoot, S., and J. A. Olson. 1974. Plasma and liver concentrations of vitamin A in a normal population of urban Thai. Am. J. Clin. Nutr. 27:883–891.

Temperley, I. J., M. J. M. Meehan, and P. B. B. Gatenby. 1968. Serum folic acid levels in pregnancy and their relationship to megaloblastic marrow change. Br. J. Haematol. 14:13–19.

Theuer, R. C. 1972. Effect of oral contraceptive agents on vitamin and mineral needs: a review. J. Reprod. Med. 8:13–19.

Thompson, J. N., P. Erdody, and W. B. Maxwell. 1973. Simultaneous fluorometric determinations of vitamins A and E in human serum and plasma. Biochem. Med. 8:403–414.

Tripathy, K. 1968. Erythrocyte transketolase activity and thiamine transfer across human placenta. Am. J. Clin. Nutr. 21:739–742.

Turton, C. W. G., T. C. B. Stamp, P. Stanley, and J. D. Maxwell. 1977. Altered vitamin D metabolism in pregnancy. Lancet 1:222–225.

Underwood, B. A. 1974. The determination of vitamin A and aspects of its distribution, mobilization and transport in health and disease. World Rev. Nutr. Dietetics 19:123–172.

U.S. Department of Health, Education, and Welfare. 1974. Preliminary Findings of the First Health and Nutrition Examination Survey, United States, 1971–1972. Dietary Intake and Biochemical Findings. DHEW Publication No. (HRA) 74-1219-1. 183 pp.

Vobecky, J. S., J. Vobecky, D. Shapcott, and L. Munan. 1974a. Vitamin C and outcome of pregnancy. Lancet I:630.

Vobecky, J. S., J. Vobecky, D. Shapcott, R. Blanchard, R. LaFond, D. Cloutier, and L. Munan. 1974b. Serum alpha-tocopherol in pregnancies with normal or pathological outcomes. Can. J. Physiol. Pharmacol. 52:384–388.

Wachstein, M. 1964. Evidence for a relative vitamin B_6 deficiency in pregnancy and some disease states. Vit. Horm. 22:705–719.

Wachstein, M., and A. Gudaitis. 1952. Disturbance of vitamin B_6 metabolism in pregnancy. J. Lab. Clin. Med. 40:550–557.

Wachstein, M. and A. Gudaitis. 1953. Disturbance of vitamin B_6 metabolism in pregnancy. II. The influence of various amounts of pyridoxine hydrochloride upon the abnormal tryptophane load test in pregnant women. J. Lab. Clin. Med. 42:98–107.

Wachstein, M., C. Moore, and L. W. Graffeo. 1957. Pyridoxal phosphate (B_6-al-PO_4) levels of circulating leukocytes in maternal and cord blood. Proc. Soc. Exp. Biol. Med. 96:326–328.

Wachstein, M., J. D. Kellner, and J. M. Ortiz. 1959. Pyridoxal phosphate in plasma and leukocytes of normal and pregnant subjects following B_6 load tests. Proc. Soc. Exp. Biol. Med. 103:350–353.

Warnock, L. G., U. Frattali, and A. M. Preston. 1975. Transketolase activity of blood hemolysate, a useful index for diagnosing thiamine deficiency. Clin. Chem. 21:432–436.

Wasserman, R. H., and R. A. Corradino. 1973. Vitamin D, calcium, and protein synthesis. Vit. Horm. 31:43–103.

Watson, J. D., and D. Y. Dako. 1975. Erythrocyte transketolase activity in adult Ghanaian subjects. Clin. Chim. Acta 59:55–61.

Waxman, S. 1975. Folate binding proteins. Br. J. Haematol. 29:23–29.

Wei Wo, C. K., and H. H. Draper. 1975. Vitamin E status of Alaskan Eskimos. Am. J. Clin. Nutr. 28:808–813.

Woodring, M. J., and C. A. Storvick. 1970. Effect of pyridoxine supplementation on glutamic-pyruvic transaminase and in vitro stimulation in erythrocytes of normal women. Am. J. Clin. Nutr. 23:1385–1395.

Yeung, D. L., and P. L. Chan. 1975. Effects of a progestogen and a sequential type oral contraceptive on plasma vitamin A, vitamin E, cholesterol and triglycerides. Am. J. Clin. Nutr. 28:686–691.

Young, J. E., C. Barrows, K. Okuda, and B. F. Chow. 1959. Vitamin B_{12} serum levels in pregnancy. Obstet. Gynecol. 14:149–153.

Yusufji, D., V. I. Mathan, and S. J. Baker. 1973. Iron, folate, and vitamin B_{12} nutrition in pregnancy: a study of 1000 women from southern India. Org. Mond. Sante W.H.O. 48:15–22.

7

Trace
Elements

K. MICHAEL HAMBIDGE
and ALVIN M. MAUER

Until very recently laboratory instrumentation and techniques have not in general been available for the assessment of trace-element nutritional status. Even today, biochemical indices for many of the "newer" trace elements are either totally lacking or are limited in their applicability to the research laboratory. Recent advances, especially in the area of analytical instrumentation, have greatly facilitated the quantitative measurement of more established elements such as zinc and copper, as well as iron, in biological samples. However, the measurement of the concentration of these elements in blood and other samples does not necessarily provide a valid index of nutritional status, and this is especially true during pregnancy. Even for zinc and copper, significant interlaboratory differences still exist for normal values. Therefore, until there is more general agreement on absolute values for norms, it is important for each individual laboratory to establish its own normal ranges.

IRON

The assessment of the nutritional status for iron during pregnancy is important because of the frequency with which a deficiency of iron leads to the development of anemia in pregnant women. There are various tests for the measurement of iron status. Bainton and Finch

157

(1964) have described the two degrees of the deficiency state for iron. Iron deficiency is taken to mean simply a reduction in total body iron; iron-deficient erythropoiesis results when there is an inadequate supply of iron to meet the needs of the erythroid marrow, ultimately causing anemia. The various tests for nutritional status for iron have varying degrees of sensitivity in defining these two departures from normal. The sensitivity of these tests in determining iron nutriture has been studied by evaluating them during the progression from iron deficiency to iron-deficient erythropoiesis (Conrad and Crosby, 1962; Bainton and Finch, 1964; and Charlton and Bothwell, 1970).

The best indicator of adequate iron stores is the presence of stainable iron in the macrophages of the bone marrow as determined by the Prussian Blue reaction on smears prepared from bone marrow aspirates. If iron stores are reduced to the point of depletion of the reticuloendothelial iron, the next events are a decrease in serum iron and an increase in the serum iron-binding capacity, leading to a decrease in the percent saturation of transferrin. Coincidental with the decline in saturation of the transferrin, the number of iron-staining granules in the developing red cells (or sideroblasts) decreases. When the saturation of transferrin is below 16 percent and that of sideroblasts less than 10 percent, both the rate of erythrocyte production and the size and hemoglobin concentration of erythrocytes decrease.

This change in erythropoiesis is first manifest by the transient development of normocytic anemia, which is followed by the characteristic microcytic hypochromic anemia of iron deficiency. The first changes in the red cell morphology consist of a decreased mean corpuscular volume (MCV) and mean corpuscular hemoglobin (MCH), followed by a decrease in the mean corpuscular hemoglobin concentration (MCHC).

There are some other measures of the state of iron nutriture as well. An increase in iron absorption from the gut can be demonstrated only with an absence of stainable iron in the bone marrow (Conrad and Crosby, 1962). A normal individual absorbs less than 10 percent of an administered dose of iron salt, but this level increases with the development of iron deficiency. The final step in the biosynthesis of heme involves the incorporation of iron into protoporphyrin. An increase in free erythrocyte protoporphyrin levels characterizes iron deficiency; levels are sixfold greater than normal in patients in whom the iron-deficiency state is characterized by an absence of stainable marrow iron (Dagg et al., 1966). These increased values, however, are seen only when the saturation of transferrin has decreased below 16 percent. Thus, this test is no more sensitive than a determination of serum iron and iron-binding capacity. Another measure of depletion of iron stores is the determination of serum ferritin (Jacobs *et al.*, 1972). The concentration becomes less than 10 ng/ml at a time when the saturation of transferrin is less than 16 percent. Thus, this method has the same significance in detecting iron deficiency as does the transferrin saturation determination.

There are special considerations that must be taken into account when applying these measures of the nutritional status for iron during pregnancy. Iron deficiency defined as a lack of iron stores is relatively common among young, nonpregnant women. Scott and Pritchard (1967) demonstrated that about one-third of apparently healthy young women without history of hemorrhage or pregnancy had negligible iron stores. In another one-third of these women, iron stores approximated only the iron content of a single unit of blood. Thus, women of child-bearing age are likely to have absent or diminished iron stores.

The iron requirements, however, of pregnancy are considerable. The term-sized infant, on the average, contains about 200 to 250 mg of iron (Sturgeon, 1956). The placenta and cord containing fetal blood contain about 50 mg of iron. The maternal red cell volume during pregnancy increases on the average about 500 ml, representing the need for an additional 500 mg of iron (DeLeeuw *et al.*, 1966; Pritchard *et al.*, 1969). Therefore, the total maternal iron requirements during pregnancy typically are from 750 to 900 mg. Regardless of the maternal status for iron nutrition, iron is transported from mother to fetus (Pritchard *et al.*, 1969).

Therefore, because of the frequency of depleted iron stores in women beginning pregnancy and the further drain on iron stores during pregnancy, the incidence of iron deficiency anemia developing late in pregnancy in women not provided an extra source of iron would be expected to be great. The criteria for distinguishing between physiological changes of pregnancy with respect to the biochemical indices of iron nutrition and the findings related to true iron deficiency must be evaluated with care. For example, reports of studies of women not given supplemental iron during pregnancy have indicated an inverse relationship between serum iron levels and the length of gestation. Serum iron values decrease as pregnancy proceeds, and, at the same time, the serum iron-binding capacity increases with a concomitant decrease in transferrin saturation. However, increase in total iron-binding capacity is characteristic of pregnancy in the mouse without iron deficiency (Jepson and Lowenstein, 1968) and occurs in healthy women receiving oral contraceptives (Burton, 1967). There is a problem, therefore, of ascribing the cause of an increasing serum iron-

binding capacity during pregnancy to endocrine effect or iron depletion. Also, the potential effect of a physiologic increase in iron-binding
capacity on the interpretation of decreasing percent saturation of
transferrin must also be determined to properly evaluate the biochemical indices of iron during pregnancy.

There are two methods by which this assessment has been accomplished. As one method of evaluating the significance of changes,
pregnant women have been given iron and serial observations subsequently made to determine the changes in serum iron, iron-binding
capacity, and percent transferrin saturation (Carr, 1974; Duke et al.,
1974). The other method of study has been the observation of women
given supplemental iron in comparison with another group in which no
supplementation was used (Hancock et al., 1968). From an evaluation
of these types of studies, it is possible to distinguish between the
normal physiological alterations of the biochemical indices of iron
nutriture and those that are associated with the progressive development of true iron deficiency during pregnancy.

Therefore, in evaluating any reports of studies of iron nutritional
status during pregnancy, it is important to know the characteristics of
the group under study. The frequency of iron depletion in women at the
beginning of pregnancy varies greatly with socioeconomic factors.
Even in those studies of women receiving supplementation it is important to note the amount of iron recommended (DeLeeuw et al., 1966)
and whether there are reasons to suspect lack of compliance with the
recommended dosage scheduled (Molina et al., 1974). In the following
presentation of data, it will be noted whether these studies were
obtained with or without effective iron supplementation.

Values for serum iron levels obtained in women with and without
iron supplementation are given in Table 7-1. Most studies of unsupplemented subjects describe a decrease in serum iron values with advancing gestation. An exception is the study by Rath et al. (1950) in women
presumed to be unsupplemented (since no mention is made of supplementation), in which are reported values similar to those obtained in
other studies in which iron supplementation was given during the
course of pregnancy. In studies in which iron supplementation was
given by either injectable iron dextran or daily oral iron, the serum iron
values do not change significantly during pregnancy. The importance
of knowing the dose of iron used for supplementation is illustrated by
the work of DeLeeuw et al. (1966), in which one group (values not
given in the Table 7-1) was given one-half of the iron supplementation
of those women shown in Table 7-1 as the supplemented group. The
women receiving half doses of supplemental iron did not develop

TABLE 7-1 Serum Iron Values (μg/dl)

References	Nonpregnant	Pregnant			Postpartum
		Early (10–20 wk)	Mid (21–29 wk)	Late (30–40 wk)	
Nonsupplemented					
Fay et al. (1949)[a]		105 (40–215)[b]	75 (30–180)	60 (20–220)	80 (50–125)
Rath et al. (1950)		111 (62–143)	117 (16–214)	102 (54–415)	97 (49–163)
Holly (1953)	103 (64–192)	103 (60)[c]	88 (30)	68 (23)	76 (30)
Morgan (1961)		115 (24–180)	90 (20–274)	95 (22–186)	
DeLeeuw et al. (1966)[a]	103.8 ± 6.16[d]	100	75	51	60
Hancock et al. (1968)[a]		110	80	55	70
Svanberg et al. (1975)		117.0 ± 7.1	80.8 ± 5.9	65.3 ± 5.5	86.6 ± 7.9
Supplemented					
Morgan (1961)		142 (89–210)	96 (54–185)	108 (37–191)	
DeLeeuw et al. (1966)[a]		107	98	95	90
Hancock et al. (1968)[a]		120	110	125	100
Svanberg et al. (1975)		125.5 ± 5.4	109.3 ± 6.5	112.4 ± 8.9	110.2 ± 7.5

[a]Derived from graphs.
[b]Values in parentheses indicate range.
[c]Single values in parentheses for Holly's data indicate minimal values.
[d]Mean ± SE.

anemia, but they did have evidences of iron depletion as indicated by bone marrow iron stains, hemoglobin mass, and mean corpuscular hemoglobin concentration at term.

The values for total iron-binding capacity in both supplemented and nonsupplemented women during pregnancy are shown in Table 7-2. In both groups the values for total iron-binding capacity increased with increasing gestation, but the values are greater in those women who did not receive iron supplementation. Thus, it appears that there is a definite effect on the levels of transferrin related to pregnancy; these levels are further increased if there is concomitant iron depletion. Once again, it is of interest that the values reported in the studies of Rath 'et al. (1950) indicate that the nutritional status of iron in the women being studied was generally good.

In Table 7-3 is shown the percent saturation of transferrin during pregnancy. There is some progressive decrease in saturation in both groups, but it is much more pronounced in those women who did not receive supplemental iron. From the studies listed in Tables 7-1 through 7-3, it seems clear that iron supplementation ameliorates or prevents the decline in serum iron, rise in iron binding capacity, and resultant fall in percent saturation seen in unsupplemented gravidas.

Bone marrow iron stores have been evaluated during pregnancy in several studies (DeLeeuw et al., 1966; Hancock et al., 1968; Svanberg et al., 1975). At the beginning of pregnancy, from 10 to 55 percent of patients were found to have depleted iron stores in the bone marrow. Obviously, the variation reflects the population under study. In women not given supplementation by the time of delivery, there was a consistent finding of absent iron stores in the bone marrow. Even in women who had supplementation during pregnancy, from one-fourth to two-thirds had depleted marrow iron stores at term. Apparently, the marrow iron stores serve as rapidly mobilized depots of iron that can become depleted even though other indicators of iron deficiency, such as decreasing serum iron values or percent saturation of transferrin, are not evident (Hancock et al., 1968; Svanberg et al., 1975). This determination, therefore, is the most sensitive of all of the methods of assessing the nutritional status for iron during pregnancy.

Iron absorption increases during pregnancy if no supplements are given (Svanberg et al., 1975). Without supplementation the values increase from an average of 6.5 percent at the beginning of pregnancy to 14.3 percent near term. At term the range of absorption in this nonsupplemented group was from 8 to 20.1 percent. There was a good relationship between the evaluation of bone marrow iron stores and the percent of iron absorption. In women who received iron supplementa-

TABLE 7-2 Total Serum Iron-Binding Capacity (μg/dl)

References	Nonpregnant	Pregnant			Postpartum
		Early (10–20 wk)	Mid (21–29 wk)	Late (30–40 wk)	
Nonsupplemented					
Fay et al. (1949)[a]		390 (260–450)[b]	550 (360–650)	600 (375–840)	400 (350–500)
Rath et al. (1950)		290 (232–350)	313 (256–423)	336 (262–474)	308 (258–381)
Morgan (1961)		395 (230–634)	457 (294–674)	530 (264–712)	
DeLeeuw et al. (1966)	313.2 ± 10.98[c]			416	
Hancock et al. (1968)[a]		430	600	610	410
Svanberg et al. (1975)		382 ± 9.3	461.2 ± 17.6	505.1 ± 19.3	346.0 ± 11.9
Supplemented					
Morgan (1961)		350 (310–408)	374 (262–531)	453 (269–640)	
DeLeeuw et al. (1966)				422	
Hancock et al. (1968)[a]		380	460	520	350
Svanberg et al. (1975)		352.5 ± 8.9	409.9 ± 11.0	458.5 ± 13.7	300.2 ± 8.9

[a]Derived from graphs.
[b]Values in parentheses indicate range.
[c]Mean ± SE.

163

TABLE 7-3 Percent Transferrin Saturation

		Pregnant		
References	Early (10–20 wk)	Mid (21–29 wk)	Late (30–40 wk)	Pospartum
Nonsupplemented				
Rath et al. (1950)	38	36	30	32
	(24–59)[a]	(18–62)	(12–46)	(18–59)
DeLeeuw et al. (1966)	30	–	11	–
Hancock et al. (1968)[b]	25	15	12	17
Svanberg et al. (1975)	31.1 ± 2.1[c]	17.8 ± 1.2	13.2 ± 1.2	26.0 ± 2.5
Supplemented				
DeLeeuw et al. (1966)	30	–	25.2	–
Hancock et al. (1968)	35	25	25	28
Svanberg et al. (1975)	35.8 ± 1.9	27.2 ± 1.8	25.4 ± 2.1	38.5 ± 3.4

[a]Values in parentheses indicate range.
[b]Derived from graphs.
[c]Mean ± SE.

164

tion during pregnancy, the mean value at the beginning of pregnancy was 6.7 percent, and near term, 8.6 percent. The range of values at term was from 2.7 to 15 percent. In those women in whom greater than 10 percent absorption was found, there was a close correlation with the depletion of marrow iron stores as indicated by hemosiderin grading. Thus, the percent of iron absorption is another fairly sensitive indicator of the state of iron nutrition during pregnancy.

Values for free erythrocyte protoporphyrin during pregnancy are given in Table 7-4. Unfortunately, there are no values for women receiving iron supplementation. The increasing values for free erythrocyte protoporphyrin in these two studies indicate the presence of iron deficiency in the women under study. The increased values persist for a much longer time after delivery than other indicators of iron deficiency. Most likely, this reflects the long survival time of red cells produced during the late stages of pregnancy, and, therefore, this indicator would not be a useful guide in assessing nutritional status after delivery. It is also somewhat slower to develop and, in general, not as sensitive an indicator of the nutritional status for iron in pregnancy.

There is only one available study of plasma ferritin determinations during pregnancy, and those studies were done at the time of delivery and compared with values in cord-blood samples (Rios *et al.,* 1975). The values in women at term ranged from 5 to 32 ng/ml. The authors divided the women into two groups, those with less than 9 ng/ml and those with greater than that level. In these two groups, other measures of iron nutriture such as hemoglobin, transferrin saturation, and the amount of iron supplementation during pregnancy were assessed. All six women having ferritin values less than 9 ng/ml had transferrin saturations less than 20 percent, with an average value of 12 percent. However, 9 women of 20 women having plasma ferritin values greater than 9 ng/ml had transferrin saturation values less than 20 percent. Thus, it would seem that the plasma ferritin value is not as sensitive an indicator of the iron nutritional status as is the transferrin saturation value.

In summary, the evaluation of bone marrow iron stores is the most sensitive indicator of the nutritional status of iron during pregnancy. Iron stores in the marrow will be depleted in some women late in pregnancy even though iron supplementation has been given and there is no evidence of iron-deficient erythropoiesis. The serum iron values during pregnancy in women receiving adequate iron supplementation should remain about constant. The total iron-binding capacity will increase even in the face of iron supplementation, but the percent

TABLE 7-4 Free Erythrocyte Protoporphyrin Values (μg/dl RBC)

References	Nonpregnant	Pregnant			Postpartum
		Early (10–20 wk)	Mid (21–29 wk)	Late (30–40 wk)	
Nonsupplemented					
Fay et al. (1949)[a]		40	42	50	50
		(10–55)[b]	(20–120)	(10–100)	
Holly (1953)	42.7	45	38.5	58	65
	(23–67)	(58)[c]	(78)	(96)	(138)

[a]Derived from graphs.
[b]Values in parentheses indicate range.
[c]Single values in parentheses for Holly's data indicate maximal values.

166

saturation of transferrin should remain greater than 20 percent. In women whose percent transferrin saturation is less than 20 percent, a response to iron treatment with a significant increase in hemoglobin and a restitution of transferrin saturation greater than 20 percent can be demonstrated (Carr, 1974). It would seem that in pregnancy, as in the nonpregnant state, a percent transferrin saturation of less than 16 percent is a good indicator of an iron deficiency state (Bainton and Finch, 1964; Charlton and Bothwell, 1970). The absorption of iron following oral administration of a radioactive test dose increases in the face of iron deficiency to greater than 10 percent; however, this is hardly a test for routine use. The determination of the free erythrocyte protoporphyrin is a later and less sensitive indicator of iron depletion. The determination of plasma ferritin values seems to be a less sensitive indicator of the nutritional status for iron than is the determination of transferrin saturation.

ZINC

Ideal biochemical indices of zinc nutritional status have not been defined. However, there are several laboratory indices of established or potential value in the assessment of zinc nutritional status and in the detection of zinc deficiency.

Plasma Zinc Concentrations

The plasma zinc concentration is currently the most widely used and accepted biochemical index of zinc nutritional status. Although hypozincemia may not be a *sine qua non* of marginal zinc deficiency, plasma zinc levels are usually depressed in human zinc deficiency. However, hypozincemia does not necessarily indicate a deficiency state: zinc levels may be depressed without a concommitant body depletion of zinc, for example, in association with acute and chronic infections, various endocrine disorders, and hypoalbuminemia.

Literature data for plasma (or serum) zinc levels during pregnancy are scanty. Results of studies in which the stage of pregnancy has been identified are summarized in Table 7-5. No details on duration of gestation were given for data included in Table 7-6. All reported mean values for plasma or serum zinc during pregnancy have been lower than those of corresponding control values for nonpregnant women. The mean level for unspecified times of gestation (Table 7-6) is 22.5 μg/100 ml (19.3 percent) lower than that of corresponding control values. Where data are available (Table 7-5), a consistent decline in

TABLE 7-5 Plasma (or Serum) Zinc Concentrations (μg/dl) during Specified Periods of Pregnancy

Reference	Type of Sample	Nonpregnant Controls, Mean ± SD		Pregnant							
				Early (10–22 wk)		Mid (23–29 wk)		Late (30–40 wk)		Postpartum (6 wk)	
		No.	Mean ± SD (or Range)	No.	Mean ± SD	No.	Mean ± SD	No.	Mean ± SD	No.	Mean ± SD
Berfenstam (1952)	Plasma		108	30	99 ± 28	18	87 ± 19	34	80 ± 17		
Hambidge and Droegemueller (1974)	Plasma	10	88 ± 8	20	68 ± 9			20	56 ± 9		
Hahn et al. (1972)	Serum	97	93					97	64		
Schraer and Calloway (1974)	Plasma							4	84	4	116
Mischel (1963)	Serum		123						109		

168

TABEL 7-6 Plasma Zinc Concentrations (µg/dl)—Duration of Pregnancy Unknown[a]

References	Type of Sample	Nonpregnant Controls			Pregnant Women			Difference in Means		Year
		No.	Mean ± SD	Range	No.	Mean ± SD	Range	µg/100 ml	%	
O'Leary and Spellacy (1969)	Plasma	27	134	95–175	30	117	96–136	−17	−12.7	1969
Halsted and Smith (1970)	Plasma	27	97 ± 11	76–112	107	63 ± 12	40–102	−34	−35.1	1970
Sinha and Gabrieli (1970)	Serum	200	120 ± 22	70–180	138	113 ± 27	64–198	−7	−6.2	1970
Rosner and Gorfien (1968)	Plasma	14	138 ± 21	87–222	27	103 ± 36	0–183	−35	−25.4	1968
Rothe (1963)	Serum		103			75		−28	−27.9	1960
Santoni et al. (1968)	Serum	10	153		10	139		−14	−9.2	1968

[a]All analyses were by atomic absorption spectrophotometry except Santoni et al. (1968).

169

mean values compared with those of nonpregnant women has been observed from wk 10 of gestation onwards. This decline appears to progress in a fairly linear fashion until wk 30 of gestation (Berfenstam, 1952). However, a more abrupt decline during the first trimester of pregnancy has been reported (Hambidge and Droegemueller, 1974). The mean value for plasma or serum zinc during late pregnancy (Table 7-5) is 27 μg/100 ml (26.5 percent) lower than that of corresponding control values.

The consistency of this decline in plasma or serum zinc levels by the last trimester of pregnancy indicates that a decline of approximately 25 percent below that of nonpregnant women is probably physiological. Factors that may contribute to this decline include the physiological increase in blood volume, a decline in serum albumin levels during the third trimester of pregnancy, and the raised levels of endogenous estrogens. Though not a consistent finding, administration of exogenous estrogens to animals (McBean et al., 1971) and man (Halsted and Smith, 1970; Prasad et al., 1975) can depress plasma zinc levels. With one exception, no details of dietary zinc intake have been given for the pregnant women included in these studies. Pregnancy is associated with increased dietary zinc requirements (Food and Nutrition Board, 1974), and there are indications that many pregnant women may not receive an optimal dietary intake of this nutrient (Sandstead, 1973). Therefore, the possibility that an inadequate dietary intake of zinc contributed to the lower levels during pregnancy cannot be excluded. However, the subjects included in one study (Schraer and Calloway, 1974) had lower plasma zinc levels in the third trimester of pregnancy than at 6 wk postpartum despite receiving a zinc-supplemented diet (the dietary zinc intake averaged 29.4 mg/day).

Data are inadequate to define a normal rate of decline of plasma zinc levels during the first and second trimesters. While it appears that a gradual decline from wk 10 of gestation onwards is probably physiological, a more abrupt decline, as reported in Hambidge and Droegemueller (1974), should not be accepted as normal without further confirmatory evidence.

The mean and range for both nonpregnant and pregnant subjects included in Tables 7-5 and 7-6 vary widely. These variations may be attributable to both sample contamination and analytical inaccuracies. Concurrently with improved methodology, normal plasma zinc levels have been revised downwards, and the generally accepted normal mean lies between 80 and 100 μg of zinc/100 ml. Values for serum zinc may be 5–15 percent higher. Because of the variation that still exists between different laboratories, the range of acceptable values during pregnancy would depend on the values for normal nonpregnant controls in the individual laboratory.

Atomic absorption spectrophotometry is now the standard analytical instrumentation for determination of plasma zinc levels. Elaborate precautions are essential to minimize the risk of sample contamination. Plastic syringes and tubes should be used for sample collection and storage. These should be checked for possible contamination. Vacutainers are not acceptable because of the high zinc content of the rubber caps.

In conclusion, mean plasma zinc levels decline gradually during the course of pregnancy. Although the decline is quite variable between individuals, plasma zinc may drop about 25 percent in normal, pregnant women. Further research is required to identify the lower limits of normalcy during late pregnancy. A provisional level of 45–50 μg/100 ml is suggested. Further research is also required to define the normal mean and range of plasma zinc levels during the first and second trimesters of pregnancy.

Hair Zinc Concentrations

Normal hair zinc levels are dependent on adequate dietary zinc intake and are depressed in human zinc deficiency. Hair zinc levels therefore provide a useful biochemical index of zinc nutritional status; however, information derived from hair analyses is retrospective. Assuming a normal rate of hair growth, the zinc content of the proximal centimeter of hair shaft adjacent to the scalp reflects the quantity of zinc taken up by the hair follicle approximately 2–6 wk previously. Thus, hair zinc determinations are of no value in the detection of current acute changes in zinc nutritional status.

Literature data on hair zinc levels during pregnancy are summarized in Table 7-7. Concentrations during the first trimester of pregnancy (Hambidge and Droegemueller, 1974) are similar to those of nonpregnant adults. The women included in this study had a small but statistically significant decline in mean hair zinc concentrations by mo 9 of gestation. This is the only report that specifies the time of gestation. The data from Baumslag *et al.* (1974) given in Table 7-7 apply only to parity-one subjects included in that study. The mean for multiparous women at term was significantly lower (mean for 17 parity-two or -three subjects = 126 μg/g; mean for 13 parity-four or greater subjects = 109 μg/g). In another study, in which hair samples were collected from Iranian women 2 days postpartum (Sarram *et al.*, 1969), hair zinc levels were noted to be dependent on economic status and quality of

TABLE 7-7 Hair Zinc Concentrations (μg of zinc/g of hair)

References	Nonpregnant Women		Early Pregnancy (10–22 wk)		Late Pregnancy (36–40 wk)		Unspecified Gestation	
	No.	Mean ± SD	No.	Mean ± SD	No.	Mean ± SD	No.	Mean ± SD
Hambidge and Droegemueller (1974)	88	180 ± 37[a]	20	171 ± 22	20	156 ± 27		–
Briggs et al. (1972)	65	198 ± 82				–	29	158 ± 85
Baumslag et al. (1974)		–			20	161[b]		158[c]
Klevay (1970)	70	167 ± 129				–	18	
Hambidge and Baum (1971)		–			20	144 ± 49[b]		–
Schroeder and Nason (1969)	47	172 ± 64				–		–

[a]From Hambidge et al. (1972) (males and females).
[b]At term.
[c]"During pregnancy and lactation."

172

the diet. Administration of oral contraceptives does not lower the zinc content of hair (Briggs *et al.*, 1972). It is probable that normal levels during pregnancy are the same as those for nonpregnant women and for young adult men (no differences related to sex have been observed), and that when lower levels are observed in late pregnancy this reflects some depletion in body zinc. Data for nonpregnant subjects are included in Table 7-7. The mean of these mean values is 179 μg of zinc/g of hair. In contrast to mean values, however, the acceptable lower limits of normalcy have not been defined. Pending clarification of this limit it is recommended that any individual value below 100 μg of zinc/g of hair be considered suggestive of inadequate zinc nutrition.

Other Biochemical Indices of Zinc Nutritional Status

The values of other biochemical indices have been less clearly defined; urine zinc excretion rates and erythrocyte zone concentrations are discussed below.

Urine Zinc Excretion Rates

The 24-h urine zinc excretion rate is depressed in severe zinc deficiency (Prasad *et al.*, 1963), but this is not a sensitive index of zinc nutritional status. The normal daily urinary zinc excretion has been reported to vary quite widely, with a range from 100 to 1,000 μg/24 h. There is conflicting evidence on the existence of a difference between men and women in urinary zinc excretion rates. As adult women may excrete less zinc in the urine than men, only data for women are included in Table 7-8. On a diet providing 15 mg of zinc per day, urinary zinc excretion rates of women taking oral contraceptives are indistinguishable from those of women not taking estrogens (J. C. King, unpublished observations). There has been only one report of urinary zinc excretion rates during pregnancy (Schraer and Calloway, 1974) (Table 7-8). The four women included in that study were receiving zinc-supplemented diets at the time, with a dietary zinc intake ranging from 28–33 mg/day. Their urinary zinc averaged 620 ± 180 μg/24 h. Though these data are insufficient to establish a normal range of urinary zinc excretion at any stage of gestation, they do suggest that rates are at least as great as those of nonpregnant women. It is tentatively concluded, therefore, that any rate during pregnancy below 100 μg of zinc/24 h is abnormally low. Rates between 100 and 150 μg of zinc/24 h should be considered "borderline."

TABLE 7-8   Urine Zinc Excretion Rates (μg Zn/24 h)

References	Nonpregnant Women		Pregnancy (Mean ± SD)		
	No.	Mean ± SD	Early	Mid	Late
Santoni et al. (1968)	10	645	–	–	–
McKenzie and Kay (1973)	105	407 ± 187	–	–	–
McKenzie (1972)	54	334 ± 168	–	–	–
Pidduck et al. (1970)	39[a]	358 ± 237	–	–	–
Hambidge (unpublished observations)	8	454 ± 218	–	–	–
Schraer and Calloway (1974)	4	–	–	–	620[b] ± 180

[a]Includes female children.
[b]Mean of 24 samples for each of four subjects.

Erythrocyte Zinc Concentrations

The red blood cell content of zinc is moderately depressed in subjects who have been chronically depleted in zinc. Most of the zinc in erythrocytes is incorporated in carbonic anhydrase and is not freely exchangeable. As the red cell has a life span of 4 mo, erythrocyte zinc levels would not be expected to decline acutely in the zinc-deficient state. Berfenstam (1952) has reported that erythrocyte zinc increases a little in the last trimester of pregnancy (1,333 ± 208 μg percent in late pregnancy compared with 1,121 ± 183 μg percent for early pregnancy). This increase has been attributed to an increase in erythrocyte carbonic anhydrase.

COPPER

In nonpregnant subjects documentation of low levels of serum copper or ceruloplasmin provides confirmatory evidence of copper depletion. Hypoproteinemia and hepatolenticular degeneration are among other causes of low serum copper and ceruloplasmin levels that have to be excluded. There are no other established biochemical indices of copper nutritional status. Ancillary data that are helpful in establishing a diagnosis of copper deficiency, but which are nonspecific, are: a hypochromic anemia which is unresponsive to iron therapy; absolute neutropenia; and X-ray evidence of osteoporosis. Documentation of copper deficiency has been limited to premature infants, cases of severe malnutrition and diarrhea rehabilitated on milk-based diets, and patients maintained on prolonged parenteral hyperalimentation.

Serum Copper Concentrations

An increase in serum copper levels during pregnancy has been a consistent finding (Table 7-9). However, reports differ considerably with respect to the magnitude of this increase. It is unlikely that these differences are explicable on the basis of variations in analytical techniques, as values for nonpregnant controls are generally quite similar. The wide variation in means may be attributable to the very large differences observed between different individuals, even at the same stage of gestation. The latter may also explain the discrepancies between different reports on the rate and stage of gestation at which copper levels increase. It should be noted that for any individual report, the data on changes in serum copper with month of pregnancy have not been derived from serial measurements on the same subjects. In addition to the rate of increase shown in Table 7-9, data have been presented in graphic form only in several other reports (Fay *et al.*, 1949; Dokumov, 1968; Schenker *et al.*, 1969; Burrows and Pekala, 1971; Hahn *et al.*, 1972). In most instances, a substantial increase has been observed by the second month of pregnancy, followed by a steady increase until term, with values returning to nonpregnant levels by 1–3 mo postpartum (Friedman *et al.*, 1969; Schenker *et al.*, 1969). However, in one report mean levels peaked at 25 wk gestation, and in other instances relatively large rates of increase have been reported in the third trimester. Increases in serum copper with duration of pregnancy may be more linear in the same individuals (O'Leary *et al.*, 1966), or when a correction factor is applied for hemodilution (De Jorge *et al.*, 1965). In Nigeria (Olatunbosun *et al.*, 1974), no increase in mean serum copper levels was observed until mo 5 of pregnancy, and values for later pregnancy were low in comparison with other reports. The authors considered that these anomalous findings may be explained by abnormalities of serum proteins that are common in that particular population.

Relatively low serum copper levels for any particular stage of gestation have been observed in association with placental insufficiency and intrauterine death (Heukenskjold and Hedenstedt, 1962; O'Leary *et al.*, 1966; Borglin and Heukenskjold, 1967; Friedman *et al.*, 1969; O'Leary, 1969; Schenker *et al.*, 1969). Indeed, serum copper levels may be of prognostic value in cases of threatened abortion.

While serum copper levels during pregnancy are certainly higher than in the nonpregnant state and in general vary directly with the duration of pregnancy, the wide variation between individuals and different studies makes it difficult to define a normal range for any

TABLE 7-9 Serum Copper Levels (μg/100 ml) by Month of Pregnancy

References	Nonpregnant Women	Month of Pregnancy									
		1	2	3	4	5	6	7	8	9	10
De Jorge et al. (1965)[a]	108 ± 8	145 ± 8	153 ± 10	200 ± 12	247 ± 28	301 ± 37	322 ± 41	356 ± 33	386 ± 25	410 ± 17	–
Friedman et al. (1969)[a]	121 (114–128)[c]	–	223 (140–265)	246 (215–260)	255 (228–293)	276 (128–300)	288 (260–316)	290 (272–340)	302 (282–355)	305 (280–365)	–
Borglin and Heuken-skjold (1967)[a]	–	–	–	172 ± 31	187 ± 46	219 ± 35	222 ± 36	236 ± 27	242 ± 69	273 ± 44	–
Hankiewicz and Sevecek (1974)[b]	109 ± 12	–	160 ± 40	167 ± 33	191 ± 24	194 ± 35	208 ± 32	208 ± 31	214 ± 22	213 ± 25	234 ± 28
von Studnitz and Berezin (1958)[b]	–	–	131	131	173	199	193	209	215	220	213

[a]Calendar months.
[b]Lunar months.
[c]Values in parentheses indicate range.

176

stage of gestation. The values given in Table 7-10 are derived from the lowest and highest values for any month of pregnancy (De Jorge *et al.*, 1965; Borglin and Heukenskjold, 1967; Friedman *et al.*, 1969; Hankiewicz and Sevecek, 1974). The majority of the lowest values were derived from Hankiewicz and Sevecek (1974), and the highest from De Jorge *et al.* (1965). These should not be regarded as definitive values for the extremes of the normal range at any stage of pregnancy. Moreover, values below the lower of these limits are more likely to reflect placental insufficiency than copper deficiency. The latter has never been documented in any normal pregnant or nonpregnant adult. However, serum copper levels do not fall below normal nonpregnant values as a result of placental dysfunction. Thus, any level below the normal range for nonpregnant women, in the absence of hypoproteinemia, would be strongly indicative of copper deficiency or an abnormality of copper metabolism. Copper levels during pregnancy are not dependent on age, race, or parity.

The recommended standard methodology for measurement of serum copper concentrations is by atomic absorption spectrophotometry.

The increase in serum copper during pregnancy is attributable, at least in large part, to the increase in endogenous estrogens (Evans, 1973) (see section on ceruloplasmin). Increased progesterone levels may also contribute to the increase (Sato and Henkin, 1973).

Serum Ceruloplasmin Concentrations

Ceruloplasmin is a glycoprotein with a molecular weight of 160,000 that contains 0.32 percent copper (eight copper atoms per molecule). In nonpregnant subjects more than 90 percent of the serum copper is ceruloplasmin copper. There are relatively few reports of serum ceruloplasmin levels during pregnancy, but a consistent increase has been observed (Markowitz *et al.*, 1955; Adelstein *et al.*, 1956; Abood and Lipman, 1965; De Jorge *et al.*, 1965; O'Reilly and Loncin, 1967; Burrows and Pekala, 1971). Early reports (Markowitz *et al.*, 1955; Adelstein *et al.*, 1956) indicated that this increase in serum ceruloplasmin was proportional to the increase in serum copper. Other data have been reported only in graphic form (Abood and Lipman, 1965; Burrows and Pekala, 1971), lack corresponding copper values (Abood and Lipman, 1965; O'Reilly and Loncin, 1967), or have been recorded only in terms of optical density (Adelstein *et al.*, 1956; Abood and Lipman, 1965). In only one study have values been reported for each month of pregnancy (De Jorge *et al.*, 1965); these values are relatively low and do not accord well with corresponding copper levels. Available data for

TABLE 7-10 Additional Data on Serum Copper Levels (μg/100 ml) during Pregnancy

References	Nonpregnant Women	Pregnancy			Unspecified Time of Gestation	Postpartum (6–11 wk)
		Early	Mid	Late		
O'Leary et al. (1966)	128 ± 12	195 ± 41	239 ± 46	261 ± 74		
Hambidge and Droegemueller (1974)	107 ± 23	162 ± 27		192 ± 24		
Lahey et al. (1953)	109 ± 17			222 ± 38		
Markowitz et al. (1955)	108 ± 9			257 ± 38		
Thompson and Watson (1949)	106 ± 18	184	221	243		119
Sinha and Gabrieli (1970)	123 ± 23			227 ± 50		
Johnson (1961)	116	203		245		
O'Leary and Spellacy (1969)	142 (104–168)[a]				231 (139–510)[a]	
Halsted and Smith (1970)	119 ± 20				249 ± 52	

[a]Range.

178

serum ceruloplasmin levels during late pregnancy are summarized in Table 7-11. In addition, a mean value of 91 ± 12.6 mg/100 ml has been reported for 10 women at term (Henkin *et al.*, 1971). The wide variation between means is of the same order of magnitude as that for serum copper levels in the third trimester (Tables 7-9 and 7-10). These data are inadequate and too variable for a definition of a normal range at any stage of gestation.

The increase in serum ceruloplasmin during pregnancy is attributable to raised levels of endogenous estrogens that induce *de novo* synthesis of ceruloplasmin in the liver (Evans *et al.*, 1970; Evans, 1973). A similar marked increase in serum ceruloplasmin occurs in subjects taking estrogen-containing oral contraceptives (Lahey *et al.*, 1953; Russ and Raymunt, 1956; Johnson *et al.*, 1959; Carruthers *et al.*, 1966; Tovey and Lathe, 1968). In turn, the increased synthesis of ceruloplasmin accounts for the increase in serum copper levels. This increase during pregnancy may represent an attempt to ensure both copper and iron transport to the developing fetus. Ceruloplasmin (ferroxidase I) has a vital function in iron mobilization.

Recommended methodology for determination of serum ceruloplasmin is either by: (1) measurement of diamine oxidase activity, preferably using para-phenylene diamine as substrate (O'Brien *et al.*, 1962), or (2) radial immunodiffusion.

Ideally, a biochemical index of copper nutritional status is required that is not affected by hormonal changes during pregnancy. Such an indicator has not as yet been identified.

CHROMIUM

Biochemical indices of chromium nutritional status that are suitable for routine application have not been established. This is in part due to the considerable difficulties of chromium analysis in biological materials that have not yet been completely resolved. However, recent research has led to the identification of several indicators of potential value. These include chromium concentrations in blood, plasma, and hair, and urinary excretion rates for this metal. It should be emphasized that these indices are currently of research interest only and are of no value to the practicing obstetrician.

Plasma Chromium Concentrations

Fasting or random plasma chromium levels have been considered not to reflect chromium nutritional status (Levine *et al.*, 1968; Mertz and

TABLE 7-11 Serum Ceruloplasmin and Copper Concentrations

References	Methodology	Nonpregnant Controls, Serum Ceruloplasmin (mg/100 ml)	Late Pregnancy, Serum Ceruloplasmin (mg/100 ml)	Late Pregnancy, Serum Copper (μg/100 ml)
Markowitz et al. (1955)	Immunologic	34 ± 4	84 ± 15	257 ± 38
De Jorge et al. (1965)	Oxidase (p-phenylenediamine)	32 ± 3.4	64 ± 7.4	410 ± 17
von Studnitz and Berezin (1958)	Oxidase (p-phenylenediamine)	28 ± 6[a]	41 ± 6.9	–
O'Leary et al. (1966)	Radial immunodiffusion	–	70–80[b]	260–280[b]

[a]Postpartum (6 wk).
[b]Approximate from graph.

Roginski, 1971; Hambidge, 1974a). However, results of two recent studies (Davidson and Burt, 1973; Pekarek *et al.*, 1975) suggest that chromium depletion may depress the fasting plasma chromium concentration and that this is detectable if the analytical technique employed is sufficiently sensitive and precise. One center has reported (Burt and Davidson, 1973; Davidson and Burt, 1973) finding lower fasting chromium concentrations in pregnant women than in nonpregnant controls (Table 7-12). Pregnancy may frequently be associated with significant depletion of maternal chromium, and a depression in plasma chromium probably reflects impairment of chromium nutritional status rather than an acceptable physiological change. Despite recent improvements in analytical methodology, large differences in mean plasma chromium concentrations (ranging from approximately 1 ng/ml (Pekarek *et al.*, 1975) to 5 ng/ml or higher (Davidson and Burt, 1973) still exist between different laboratories. Concentrations of 1 or 2 orders of magnitude higher than those shown here have been reported in the past; probably they can be explained on the basis of analytical methodology. Thus no normal range can be given that would be generally applicable to all laboratories.

The biologically potent fraction of the plasma chromium is probably a nicotinic acid-chromium complex (Mertz *et al.*, 1974) termed the glucose-tolerance factor (GTF-chromium) (Mertz, 1969). Part of the disparity in plasma chromium concentrations between different laboratories may be attributable to variable loss of GTF-chromium, depending on the analytical procedure. There are no established methods for measuring the GTF-chromium fraction of the total plasma chromium. GTF-chromium is released into the circulation from a body pool in response to increased circulating insulin. This may lead to a detectable increase in total plasma chromium following a glucose load. However, some investigators have noted a decline rather than an increase in plasma chromium following administration of oral or intravenous glucose. In these circumstances, in addition to an increase in the release of GTF-chromium into the circulation, there will also be increased peripheral utilization. The net result is presumably dependent on the relative magnitude of these two processes. Because of the difficulties in interpretation of results and the cumbersome nature of this test, it is not applicable outside the research laboratory. However, it should be noted that the plasma chromium "response" to glucose loading during the last month of pregnancy has been reported to be different from that of nonpregnant women (Hambidge, 1971; Davidson and Burt, 1973; Hambidge and Droegemueller, 1974).

TABLE 7-12 Chromium Concentrations in Plasma, Hair, and Urine

| References | Nonpregnant (Nulliparous) | | Pregnancy | | | | | | | | Parous Women | |
| | No. | Mean ± SD (Range) | Early | | Mid | | Late | | At Term | | No. | Mean ± SD |
			No.	Mean ± SD	No.	Mean ± SD (Range)	No.	Mean ± SD	No.	Mean ± SD (Range)		
Plasma chromium (ng/ml)												
Burt and Davidson (1973)	14	5.7 ± 1.1 (4.1–7.3)	21			2.9 ± 1.0 (1.3–5.9)[a]			21	2.5 ± 0.1 (1.7–3.9)		
Davidson and Burt (1973)	10	4.7 ± 0.5					10	3.0 ± 0.3				
Hambidge and Droegemueller (1974)			20	3.4 ± 1.8			20	4.0 ± 1.3				
Hair chromium (μg/g)												
Burt and Davidson (1973)	39	0.57 ± 0.37 (0.18–1.36)							37	0.36 ± 0.18 (0.11–0.72)		
Hambidge and Droegemueller (1974)			20	0.20 ± 0.19			20	0.16 ± 0.19				
Hambidge and Rodgerson (1969)	10	0.75[b] (0.20–2.81)									11	0.22 (0.04–1.14)
Urine chromium excretion (μg/24 h)												
Mitman et al. (1975)	9	7.2 ± 1.2 (5.9–10.0)										

[a] 8–38 wk of gestation.
[b] Geometric mean.

182

Hair Chromium Concentrations

The chromium content of hair appears to be dependent on chromium nutritional status (Mertz, 1969; Hambidge and Droegemueller, 1974). Hair chromium levels in pregnant women at term (Burt and Davidson, 1973; Gürson *et al.*, 1975) are lower than those of nonpregnant nulliparous women (Table 7-12), and parous women have also been found to have lower levels than nulliparous controls (Hambidge and Rodgerson, 1969). These changes have been considered to reflect impaired chromium nutritional status resulting from the increased demands of pregnancy. Thus, an acceptable range for hair chromium content during pregnancy is the same as that for nulliparous women. Again, absolute figures currently depend on the individual laboratory, and considerable geographic differences may exist (Gürson *et al.*, 1975). Therefore, lower limits of normal have not been clearly defined.

Urine Chromium Excretion

The kidneys are the major excretory route for chromium, and measurements of the rate of urinary excretion of this metal provide the most promising biochemical index of chromium nutritional status. In contrast to plasma chromium, most urinary chromium is in the "free" dialyzable form with a low molecular weight (Collins *et al.*, 1961). Though not proven, it is probable that a substantial proportion of this chromium is GTF-chromium or a metabolic product. Thus, it appears to offer a good indirect means of assessing the body status with respect to biopotent chromium. Measurement of the urinary output of this metal in response to a glucose load may be even more informative (Mitman *et al.*, 1975). There are no published data on urinary chromium excretion rates during pregnancy. Data for young, healthy, nulliparous women, whose chromium nutritional status was considered adequate, are included in Table 7-12 (Mitman *et al.*, 1975). Chromium concentrations in urine and daily excretion rates, like hair levels, are subject to considerable geographic variations (Gürson *et al.*, 1975).

Chromium at physiological levels in biological samples can be measured by atomic absorption spectrophotometry. Use of a graphite furnace is essential to achieve the sensitivity required. Though not a universal practice, careful removal of organic matter (e.g., in a low-temperature asher) appears to be important prior to introduction of the sample into the furnace (Wolf *et al.*, 1974).

Further research is necessary to establish reliable laboratory criteria for the identification of chromium deficiency. In particular, adequate methods are needed for the assessment of the body status with respect to biopotent GTF-chromium.

IODINE

Pregnancy is associated with major changes in iodine metabolism. These physiological changes complicate the evaluation of iodine nutritional status. Radioiodine tests are contraindicated during pregnancy and this further increases the difficulty of determining the iodine nutritional status of individual subjects.

The most widely used biochemical index of iodine nutritional status is the 24-h urine iodine excretion rate or the urine iodine:creatinine ratio (Follis, 1964; Underwood, 1971). The kidney is the major excretory route for iodine, and urine iodine excretion rates are dependent on dietary intake of this element. This test is particularly valuable for population surveys, but less reliable for the individual subject; the latter is attributable in part to variations in the renal clearance of iodine. In nonpregnant subjects, a urine iodine excretion of less than 40 μg/24 h is suggestive of iodine deficiency (Underwood, 1971). Mean values for goitrous areas range from 8.6–41.2 μg/24 h. In nongoitrous areas means range from 72–343 μg/24 h with an overall mean of 150 μg/24 h (Riggs, 1952). Wayne et al. (1964) reported an individual range of 44–171 in the United Kingdom. There are very few data on urine iodine excretion rates during pregnancy, and it is unclear whether the same lower limits of normal apply, especially as the renal clearance of iodine is approximately doubled during pregnancy (Aboul-Khair et al., 1964; Aboul-Khair and Crooks, 1965). However, the normal absolute excretion rate is generally considered to be similar to that of nonpregnant subjects (Hytten and Lind, 1973). A normal group of euthyroid pregnant women in Lima, Peru, had a mean urinary excretion rate of 182 μg of iodine/24 h (Pretell et al., 1974) at unspecified times of gestation. A mean value excretion rate of 146 μg/24 h has been reported for both mid- and late pregnancy (Dworkin et al., 1966); corresponding values for the same five subjects at 1 and 2 mo postpartum were 153 and 131 μg/24 h, respectively. There are unconfirmed suggestions that the excretion rate may be increased during the last month of gestation (Enright et al., 1935; Puppel and Curtis, 1938). In a goitrous area the mean urinary excretion during pregnancy was 31 μg of iodine/24 h (Pretell et al., 1974); this is similar to findings for nonpregnant subjects in such areas.

The urine iodine is almost entirely inorganic and is derived from the plasma inorganic iodide (PII). The concentration of PII is very low (approximately 0.2 μg/100 ml) and is difficult to measure directly (Aboul-Khair and Crooks, 1965). The PII can be determined indirectly with radioiodine studies (PII = urinary I $\times$ [132]I plasma/[132]I urine), but such tests are contraindicated during pregnancy. The rate of urine iodine excretion correlates well with the PII if renal clearance of iodine is "normal." The PII is unusually low in pregnancy, presumably at least in part due to the increased renal clearance. To compensate for the low PII, thyroid clearance of iodine is increased two- to threefold to a rate of approximately 50 ml/min in order to achieve the same absolute iodine uptake by the thyroid in unit time (approximately 2 μg/h) as in nonpregnant subjects (Aboul-Khair and Crooks, 1965). The increased thyroid clearance of iodine will in turn accentuate the depression of PII levels. Thus, levels of PII and thyroid clearance rates that are diagnostic of iodine deficiency in the nonpregnant state must be considered normal during pregnancy.

Tests of thyroid function may be affected by iodine deficiency; e.g., serum thyroxine (T4) and triiodothyronine (T3) can be reduced, and plasma thyrostimuline (TSH) levels can be increased. In pregnancy, there is an estrogen-stimulated increase in thyroid-binding globulin (TBG) levels to approximately twice normal nonpregnant levels (Table 7-13). This increase in thyroxine (T4)-binding capacity necessitates an increase in total T4 to ensure maintenance of the normal small, but physiologically important, fraction of free T4 in the serum. This is achieved by the negative feedback to the pituitary provided by a decrease in the T4, which leads to the release of increased TSH; in turn, this results in increased T4 production and release, the major part binding to the TBG. Thus, in pregnancy there is an increase in TSH and total T4 levels are elevated to a mean of approximately 2.5 μg/100 ml above nonpregnant levels; T3 levels are also elevated during pregnancy. Free thyroxine levels are maintained within the lower limits of the normal nonpregnant range (Table 7-13). The increase in TBG is detectable by wk 3 after ovulation, and the increase in T4 has been reported early in the first trimester. The increases are quite sharp and rapidly reach a plateau for the remainder of pregnancy. However, there are wide individual variations in T4 that overlap the nonpregnant range.

Determination of urine iodine is accomplished by a chloric acid digestion followed by use of the cerium-arsenic catalytic system to measure iodine (Zak *et al.,* 1952; Benotti and Benotti, 1963). The rate of urine excretion of creatinine increases during pregnancy. If estimations of 24-h urine iodine excretion are based on measurements of the urine iodine:creatinine ratio (Vought and London, 1965), the increase

TABLE 7-13 Changes in Selected Thyroid Function Tests during Pregnancy

References	Test	Nonpregnant Controls	Pregnancy			Postpartum
			Early	Mid	Late	
Aboul-Khair and Crooks (1965); Mestman et al. (1969); Lemarchand-Beraud and Mean (1970); Hallman et al. (1951)	Serum thyroxine (µg/100 ml)	4.7–6.3[a] (3–8)[b]	6.9–7.8 (4–14)	6.9–10.2 (4–14)	7.8–10.2 (4–14)	4.1–5.4 (3.0–6.3)
Man et al. (1969)[a]	PBI					
	BEI		7.1 (±1.0)[c]	7.6 (±1.0)	7.6 (±0.9)	5.0 (±0.9)
Mestman et al. (1969)	T₄(c)	(2.9–6.4)		6.8	6.8	4.3
Souma et al. (1973); Malkasian and Mayberry (1970)	T₄(d)	5.8–6.8 (4–9.4)	7.7–9.8 (6–18)	(4.1 ± 9.6) 8.4–9.9 (4.5–14)	(4.1 ± 9.6) 8.6–9.9 (4.5–14)	(2.4 ± 6.2) 5.9
Lemarchand-Beraud and Mean (1970); Souma (1973); Malkasian and Mayberry (1970)	Free thyroxine (ng/100 ml)	1.5–4.4	1.2–4.3	1.1–3.9	1.6–4.1	
Man et al. (1969)	TBG (µg%)	22 (18–25)		56 (±6.2)	56 (±6.2)	26 (±3.6)
Malkasian and Mayberry (1970)	TSH (uu/ml)	8.3 (±3.9)	12.8 (±3.4)	11.1 (±3.8)	7.6 (±2.5)	8.5 (±2.7)
Fisher et al. (1973); Eastman et al. (1973); Lieblich and Utiger (1973)	Serum tri-iodo-thyronine (ng/100 ml)	(70–160)	–	179 (152–224)	156–209 (144–288)	

[a] Range of means for cited reports.
[b] Examples of individual range of values.
[c] One standard deviation.

186

in creatinine excretion should be taken into consideration when computing the total 24-h excretion. However, it is preferable to collect a 24-h sample. Radioimmunoassay procedures are the ideal method for measuring thyroxine [T4(D) and T4(RIA)] and triiodothyronine [T3(RIA)]. Data for T4 derived from measurement of the protein-bound iodine (PBI), butanol-extractable iodine (BEI), and the resin column absorption technique [T4(C)] are included in Table 7-13. Though theoretically less ideal, mean results obtained with these techniques are similar to those for T4(D). Fisher (1973) has recently reviewed laboratory techniques used in the investigation of thyroid function.

In summary, there is a need to define the lower acceptable limits of normal for urine iodine excretion rates during pregnancy. Interpretation of T3 and T4 levels is difficult because of the wide range of individual levels and their dependence on factors other than iodine nutritional status. However, unusually low values of serum total T4, T3, and/or free T4 can be valuable in the diagnosis of iodine deficiency. In pregnant women resident in an endemic goitrous area, iodine supplementation was found to increase total and free T4 levels and to lower TSH levels (Pretell *et al.*, 1974).

MANGANESE

There has been only one report of manganese concentrations in blood plasma and hair of pregnant women (Table 7-14) (Hambidge and Droegemueller, 1974). There is no information on the manganese nutritional status of these women. The values in Table 7-14 are similar to levels for adult men and nonpregnant women in the same laboratory. Differences between the first and third trimester are not statistically significant for either hair or plasma manganese concentrations. It is not

TABLE 7-14   Plasma and Hair Manganese Levels during Pregnancy

Test	Nonpregnant controls[b]	Pregnancy[a]		
		Early	Mid	Late
Plasma (ng/ml)		1.4 ± 0.9	–	2.0 ± 0.9
Hair (μg/g)	0.29 ± 0.13	0.17 ± 0.21	–	0.13 ± 0.13

[a]Data from Hambidge and Droegemueller (1974).
[b]Data from Hambidge *et al.* (1974).

known if either plasma or hair manganese levels provide valid biochemical indices of manganese nutritional status.

OTHER TRACE ELEMENTS

Other trace elements of recognized nutritional importance in animals or man include: molybdenum, selenium, cobalt, fluorine, nickel, silicon, vanadium, and tin. Useful biochemical indices for these elements have not been established.

REFERENCES

Abood, L. G., and V. C. Lipman. 1965. Blood ceruloplasmin activity during human pregnancy with special reference to Tay-Sachs disease. Am. J. Obstet. Gynecol. 92:529–533.

Aboul-Khair, S. A., and J. Crooks. 1965. A comparative study of iodine metabolism in pregnancy, sporadic goitre and thyrotoxicosis. Acta Endocrinol. 48:14–22.

Aboul-Khair, S. A., J. Crooks, A. C. Turnbull, and F. E. Hytten. 1964. The physiological changes in thyroid function during pregnancy. Clin. Sci. 27:195–207.

Adelstein, S. J., T. L. Coombs, and B. L. Vallee. 1956. Metalloenzymes and myocardial infarction. I. The relation between serum copper and ceruloplasmin and its catalytic activity. N. Engl. J. Med. 255:105–109.

Bainton, F. B., and C. A. Finch. 1964. The diagnosis of iron deficiency anemia. Am. J. Med. 37:62–70.

Baumslag, N., Yeager, D., Levin, L., and H. G. Petering. 1974. Trace metal content of maternal and neonate hair. Arch. Environ. Health 29:186–191.

Benotti, J., and N. Benotti. 1963. Protein-bound iodine, total iodine, and butanol-extractable iodine by partial automation. Clin. Chem. 9:408–411.

Berfenstam, R. 1952. Studies on blood zinc. A clinical and experimental investigation into the zinc content of plasma and blood corpuscles with special reference to infancy. Acta Paediatr. Suppl. 87:41–45.

Borglin, N. E., and F. Heukenskjold. 1967. Studies on serum copper in pregnancy. Acta Obstet. Gynecol. Scand. 46:119–125.

Briggs, M. H., M. Briggs, and A. Wakatama. 1972. Trace elements in human hair. Experientia 28:406–407.

Burrows, S., and B. Pekala. 1971. Serum copper and ceruloplasmin in pregnancy. Am. J. Obstet. Gynecol. 109:907–909.

Burt, R. L., and I. W. F. Davidson. 1973. Carbohydrate metabolism in pregnancy: a possible role of chromium. Acta Diabetol. Lat. 10:770–778.

Burton, J. L. 1967. Effect of oral contraceptives on haemoglobin, packed-cell volume, serum-iron, and total iron-binding capacity in healthy women. Lancet 1:978–980.

Carr, M. C. 1974. The diagnosis of iron deficiency in pregnancy. Obstet. Gynecol. 43:15–21.

Carruthers, M. E., C. B. Hobbs, and R. L. Warren. 1966. Raised serum copper and caeruloplasmin levels in subjects taking oral contraceptives. J. Clin. Pathol. 19:498–500.

Charlton, R. W., and T. H. Bothwell. 1970. Iron deficiency anemia. Semin. Hematol. 7:67–85.

Collins, R. J., P. O. Fromm, and W. D. Collings. 1961. Chromium excretion in the dog. Am. J. Physiol. 201:795–798.

Conrad, M. E., and W. H. Crosby. 1962. The natural history of iron deficiency induced by phlebotomy. Blood 20:173–185.

Dagg, J. H., A. Goldbert, and A. Lochhead. 1966. Value of erythrocyte protoporphyrin in the diagnosis of latent iron deficiency (Sideropenia). Br. J. Haematol. 12:326–330.

Davidson, I. W. F., and R. L. Burt. 1973. Physiologic changes in plasma chromium of normal and pregnant women: effect of a glucose load. Am. J. Obstet. Gynecol. 116:601–608.

De Jorge, F. B., D. Delascio, and M. L. Antunes. 1965. Copper and copper oxidase concentrations in the blood serum of normal pregnant women. Obstet. Gynecol. 26:225–227.

DeLeeuw, N. K. M., L. Lowenstein, and Y. Hsieh. 1966. Iron deficiency and hydremia in normal pregnancy. Medicine 45:291–315.

Dokumov, S. I. 1968. Serum copper and pregnancy. Am. J. Obstet. Gynecol. 101:217–222.

Duke, A. B., J. Kelleher, B. B. Bauminger, and G. Walters. 1974. Serum iron and iron binding capacity after total dose infusion of iron-dextran for iron deficiency anemia in pregnancy. J. Obstet. Gynaecol. Br. Commonw. 81:895–900.

Dworkin, H. J., J. A. Jacquez, and W. H. Beierwaltes. 1966. Relationship of iodine ingestion to iodine excretion in pregnancy. J. Clin. Endocrinol. Metab. 26:1329–1342.

Eastman, C. J., J. M. Corcoran, A. Jequier, R. P. Ekins, and E. S. Williams. 1973. Triiodothyronine concentration in cord and maternal sera at term. Clin. Sci Mol. Med. 45:251–255.

Enright, L., V. V. Cole, and F. A. Hitchcock. 1935. Basal metabolism and iodine excretion during pregnancy. Am. J. Physiol. 113:221–227.

Evans, G. W. 1973. Copper homeostasis in the mammalian system. Physiol. Rev. 53:535–570.

Evans, G. W., N. F. Cornatzer, and W. E. Cornatzer. 1970. Mechanism for hormone induced alterations in serum ceruloplasmin. Am. J. Physiol. 218:613–615.

Fay, J., G. E. Cartwright, and M. M. Wintrobe. 1949. Studies on free erythrocyte protoporphyrin, serum iron, serum iron-binding capacity and plasma copper during normal pregnancy. J. Clin. Invest. 28:487–491.

Fielding, J., M. C. O'Shaughnessy, and G. M. Brunstrom. 1965. Iron deficiency without anaemia. Lancet 2:9–12.

Fisher, D. A. 1973. Advances in the laboratory diagnosis of thyroid disease, part 1. J. Pediatr. 82:1–9.

Fisher, D. A., J. H. Dussault, C. J. Hobel, and R. Lam. 1973. Serum and thyroid gland triiodothyronine in the human fetus. Clin. Endocrinol. Metab. 36:397–400.

Follis, R. H., Jr. 1964. Patterns of urinary iodine excretion in goitrous and nongoitrous areas. Am. J. Clin. Nutr. 14:253–268.

Food and Nutrition Board (National Research Council). 1974. Recommended Dietary Allowances, 8th rev. ed. National Academy of Sciences, Washington, D.C., 129 pp.

Friedman, S., C. Bahary, B. Eckerling, and B. Gans. 1969. Serum copper level as an index of placental function. Obstet. Gynecol. 33:189–194.

Gürson, C. T., G. Saner, W. Mertz, W. R. Wolf, and S. Söpücü. 1975. Nutritional significance of chromium in different chronological age groups and in populations differing in nutritional background. Nutr. Rep. Int., 12:9–17.

Hahn, N., K. Paschen, and J. Haller. 1972. Das verhalten von kupfer. Eisen. Magnesium. Calcium und zink bei frauen mit normalem menstruation-scyclus unter einnahme von ovulationshemmern und in der graviditat. Arch. Gynaekol., 213:176–186.

Hallman, B. L., P. K. Bondy, and M. A. Hagewood. 1951. Determination of serum protein-bound iodine as a routine clinical procedure. Arch. Intern. Med. 87:817–824.

Halsted, J. A., and Smith, J. C., Jr. 1970. Plasma-zinc in health and disease. Lancet i:322–324.

Hambidge, K. M. Unpublished observations.

Hambidge, K. M. 1971. Chromium nutrition in the mother and the growing child, pp. 169–194. In W. Mertz and W. E. Cornatzer, eds., Newer Trace Elements in Nutrition. Marcel Dekker, Inc., New York.

Hambidge, K. M. 1974a. Chromium nutrition in man. Am. J. Clin. Nutr. 27:505–514.

Hambidge, K. M. 1974b. The clinical significance of trace element deficiencies in man. Proc. Nutr. Soc. 33:249–255.

Hambidge, K. M., and D. Baum. 1971. Chromium, iron, zinc and magnesium concentrations in newborn hair. Clin. Res. 19:220.

Hambidge, K. M., and W. Droegemueller. 1974. Changes in plasma and hair concentrations of zinc, copper, chromium, and manganese during pregnancy. Obstet. Gynecol. 44:666–672.

Hambidge, K. M., and D. O. Rodgerson. 1969. Comparison of hair chromium levels of nulliparous and parous women. Am. J. Obstet. Gynecol. 103:320–321.

Hambidge, K. M., C. Hambidge, M. Jacobs, and J. D. Baum. 1972. Low levels of zinc in hair, anorexia, poor growth, and hypogeusia in children. Pediatr. Res. 6:868–874.

Hambidge, K. M., P. Walravens, V. Kumar, and C. Tuchinda. 1974. Chromium, zinc, manganese, copper, nickel, iron and cadmium concentrations in the hair of residents of Chandigarh, India and Bangkok, Thailand, p. 39. In D. D. Hemphill, ed., Trace Substances in Environmental Health, vol. VIII. University of Missouri Press, Columbia.

Hancock, K. W., P. A. Walker, and T. A. Harper. 1968. Mobilisation of iron in pregnancy. Lancet 2:1055–1058.

Hankiewicz, V. J., and E. Sevecek. 1974. Untersuchungen uber den Kupfer und zeruloplasmingehalt bei frauen wahrend der schwangerschaft und bei solchen mit gewissen gynakologischen krankheiten. Zentralbl. Gynaekol. 96:905–909.

Henkin, R. I., R. E. Lippoldt, J. Bilstad, and H. Edelhoch. 1975. A zinc protein isolated from human parotid saliva. Proc. Natl. Acad. Sci. U.S.A. 72:488–492.

Henkin, R. I., J. R. Marshall, and S. Meret. 1971. Maternal-fetal metabolism of copper and zinc at term. Am. J. Obstet. Gynecol. 110:131–134.

Heukenskjold, F., and S. Hedenstedt. 1962. Serum copper determinations in normal pregnancy and abortion. Acta Obstet. Gynecol. Scand. 41:41–47.

Holly, R. G. 1953. The iron and iron-binding capacity of serum and the erythrocyte protoporphyrin in pregnancy. Obstet. Gynecol. 2:119–126.

Hytten, F. E., and T. Lind. 1973. Diagnostic Indices in Pregnancy, pp. 72–76. CIBA-Geigy Ltd., Basel, Switzerland.

Jacobs, A., F. Miller, M. Worwood, M. R. Beamish, and C. A. Wardrop. 1972. Ferritin in the serum of normal subjects and patients with iron deficiency and iron overload. Br. Med. J. 4:206–208.

Jepson, J., and L. Lowenstein. 1968. Hormonal control of erythropoiesis during pregnancy in the mouse. Br. J. Haematol. 14:555–562.

Johnson, N. C. 1961. Study of copper and zinc metabolism during pregnancy. Proc. Soc. Exp. Biol. Med. 108:518–519.

Johnson, N. C., T. Kheim, and W. B. Kountz. 1959. Influence of sex hormones on total serum copper. Proc. Soc. Exp. Biol. Med. 102:98–99.

Klevay, L. M. 1970. Hair as a biopsy material. I. Assessment of zinc nutriture. Am. J. Clin. Nutr., 23:284–289.

Lahey, M. E., C. J. Gubler, G. E. Cartwright, and M. M. Wintrobe. 1953. Studies on copper metabolism. VII. Blood copper in pregnancy and various pathologic states. J. Clin. Invest. 32:329–339.

Lemarchand-Beraud, T., and P. Mean. 1970. Pituitary regulation of thyroid function in pregnancy. Horm. Metab. Res. 2:338–343.

Levine, R. A., D. H. P. Streeten, and R. J. Doisy. 1968. Effects of oral chromium supplementation on the glucose tolerance of elderly human subjects. Metab. Clin. Exp. 17:114–125.

Lieblich, J. M., and R. D. Utiger. 1973. Triiodothyronine in cord serum. J. Pediatr. 82:290–292.

Lo, J. S., and J. A. Kellen. 1971. Spontaneous partial reactivation of chelated placental alkaline phosphatase in the absence of zinc. Enzyme 12:606–617.

Malkasian, G. D., and W. E. Mayberry. 1970. Serum total and free thyroxine and thyrotropin in normal and pregnant women, neonates, and women receiving progestogens. Am. J. Obstet. Gynecol. 108:1234–1238.

Man, E. B., W. A. Reid, A. E. Hellegers, and W. S. Jones. 1969a. Thyroid function in human pregnancy. II. Serum butanol-extractable iodine values of pregnant women 14 through 44 years. Am. J. Obstet. Gynecol. 103:328–337.

Man, E. B., W. A. Reid, A. E. Hellegers, and W. S. Jones. 1969b. Thyroid function in human pregnancy. III. Serum thyroxine-binding prealbumin (TBPA) and thyroxine-binding globulin (TBG) of pregnant women aged 14 through 43 years. Am. J. Obstet. Gynecol. 103:338–347.

Markowitz, H., C. J. Gubler, J. P. Mahoney, G. E. Cartwright, and M. M. Wintrobe. 1955. Studies on copper metabolism. XIV. Copper, ceruloplasmin, and oxidase activity in sera of normal human subjects, pregnant women, and patients with infection, hepatolenticular degeneration and the nephrotic syndrome. J. Clin. Invest. 34:1498–1508.

McBean, L. D., J. C. Smith, Jr., and J. A. Halsted. 1971. Effect of oral contraceptive hormones on zinc metabolism in the rat. Proc. Soc. Exp. Biol. Med. 137:543–547.

McKenzie, J. M. 1972. Urinary excretion of zinc, cadmium, sodium, potassium, and creatinine in ninety-six students. Proc. Univ. Otago Med. Sch. 50:16–18.

McKenzie, J. M., and D. L. Kay. 1973. Urinary excretion of cadmium, zinc and copper in normotensive and hypertensive women. N. Z. Med. J. 78:68–70.

Mertz, W. 1969. Chromium occurrence and function in biological systems. Physiol. Rev. 49:163–239.

Mertz, W., and E. E. Roginski. 1971. Chromium metabolism: the glucose tolerance factor, pp. 123–153. *In* W. Mertz and W. Cornatzer, ed., New Trace Elements in Nutrition. Marcel Dekker, Inc., New York.

Mertz, W., E. W. Toepfer, E. E. Roginski, and M. M. Polansky. 1974. Present knowledge of the role of chromium. Fed. Proc. 33:2275–2280.

Mestman, J. H., J. W. H. Niswonger, G. V. Anderson, and P. R. Manning. 1969. Evaluation of thyroid function during and after pregnancy. Am. J. Obstet. Gynecol. 103:322–327.

Mischel, W. 1963. Zinc metabolism in pregnancy. Med. Welt 32:1594–1600.

Mitman, F. W., W. R. Wolf., J. L. Kelsay, and E. S. Prather. 1975. Urinary chromium levels of nine young women eating freely chosen diets. J. Nutr. 105:64–68.

Molina, R. A., M. Diez-Ewald, G. Fernandez, and N. Velaquez. 1974. Nutritional anaemia during pregnancy, a comparative study of two socioeconomic classes. J. Obstet. Gynaecol. Br. Commonw. 81:454–458.

Morgan, E. H. 1961. Plasma-iron and haemoglobin levels in pregnancy. Lancet 1:9–12.

O'Brien, D., F. A. Ibbott, and D. O. Rodgerson. 1962. Laboratory Manual of Pediatric Microbiochemical Techniques, 4th ed. Harper & Row, Publishers, New York. 340 pp.

Olatunbosun, D. A., B. K. Adadevoh, and F. A. Adeniyi. 1974. Serum copper in normal pregnancy in Nigerians. J. Obstet. Gynaecol. 81:475–478.

O'Leary, J. A. 1969. Serum copper levels as a measure of placental function. Am. J. Obstet. Gynecol. 105:636–639.

O'Leary, J. A., and W. N. Spellacy. 1969. Zinc and copper levels in pregnant women and those taking oral contraceptives. Am. J. Obstet. Gynecol. 103:131–132.

O'Leary, J. A., G. S. Novalis, G. J. Vosburgh. 1966. Maternal serum copper concentrations in normal and abnormal gestations. Obstet. Gynecol. 28:112–117.

O'Reilly, S., and M. Loncin. 1967. Ceruloplasmin and 5-hydroxyindole metabolism in pregnancy. Am. J. Obstet. Gynecol. 97:8–12.

Pekarek, R. S., E. C. Hauer, E. J. Rayfield, R. W. Wannemacher, and W. R. Beisel. 1975. Relationship between serum chromium concentrations and glucose utilization in normal and infected subjects. Diabetes 24:350–353.

Pidduck, H. G., P. J. J. Wren, and D. A. P. Evans. 1970. Hyperzincuria of diabetes mellitus and possible genetical implications of this observation. Diabetes 19:240–247.

Prasad, A. S., H. H. Sandstead, A. R. Schulert, and A. S. El Rooby. 1963. Urinary excretion of zinc in patients with the syndrome of anemia, hepatosplenomegaly, dwarfism, and hypogonadism. J. Lab Clin. Med. 62:591–599.

Prasad, A. S., D. Oberleas, K. Y. Lei, K. S. Moghissi, and J. C. Stryker. 1975. Effect of oral contraceptive agents on nutrients: 1. Minerals. Am. J. Clin. Nutr. 28:377–384.

Pretell, E. A., P. Palacios, L. Tello, M. Wan, R. D. Utiger, and J. B. Stanbury. 1974. Iodine deficiency and the maternal-fetal relationship, pp. 143–155. In J. T. Dunn and G. A. Medeiros-Neto, ed., Endemic Goiter and Cretinism: Continuing Threats to World Health. Pan American Health Organization, Washington, D.C.

Pritchard, J. A., P. J. Whalley, and D. E. Scott. 1969. The influence of maternal folate and iron deficiencies on intrauterine life. Am. J. Obstet. Gynecol. 104:388–396.

Puppel, I. D., and G. M. Curtis. 1938. Iodine balance in exophthalmic goiter. Arch. Pathol. 26:1093–1120.

Rath, C. E., W. Caton, D. E. Reid, C. A. Finch, and L. Conroy. 1950. Hematological changes and iron metabolism of normal pregnancy. Surg. Gynecol. Obstet. 90:320–396.

Riggs, D. S. 1952. Quantitative aspects of iodine metabolism in man. Pharmacol. Rev. 4:284–370.

Rios, E., D. A. Lipschitz, J. D. Cook, and N. J. Smith. 1975. Relationship of maternal and infant iron stores as assessed by determination of plasma ferritin. Pediatrics 55:694–699.

Rosner, F., and P. C. Gorfien. 1968. Erythrocyte and plasma zinc and magnesium levels in health and disease. J. Lab Clin. Med. 72:213–219.

Rothe, K. 1963. Serum zinc in normal pregnancy and in early and late toxemias. Arch. Gynaekol. 192:349–362.

Russ, E. M., and J. Raymunt. 1956. Influence of estrogens on total serum copper and caeruloplasmin. Proc. Soc. Exp. Biol. Med. 92:465–466.

Sandstead, H. H. 1973. Zinc nutrition in the United States. Am. J. Clin. Nutr. 26:1251–1260.

Santoni, G., U. Stefanini, and G. Ragni. 1968. Zinc metabolism in obstetrics. Ann. Ostet. Ginecol. 90:37–47.

Sarram, M., M. Younessi, P. Khorvash, G. A. Kfoury, and J. G. Reinhold. 1969. Zinc nutrition in human pregnancy in Fars Province, Iran. Am. J. Clin. Nutr. 22:726–732.

Sato, N., and R. I. Henkin. 1973. Pituitary-gonadal regulation of copper and zinc metabolism in the female rat. Am. J. Physiol. 225:508–512.

Schenker, J. G., E. Jungreis, and W. Z. Polishuk. 1969. Serum copper levels in normal and pathologic pregnancies. Am. J. Obstet. Gynecol. 105:933–937.

Schraer, K. K., and D. H. Calloway. 1974. Zinc balance in pregnant teenagers. Nutr. Metabol. 17:205–212.

Schroeder, H. A., and A. P. Nason. 1969. Trace metals in human hair. J. Invest. Dermatol. 53:71–78.

Scott, D. E., and J. A. Pritchard. 1967. Iron deficiency in healthy young college women. J. Am. Med. Assoc. 199:897–900.

Sinha, S. N., and E. R. Gabrieli. 1970. Serum copper and zinc levels in various pathologic conditions. Am. J. Clin. Pathol. 54:570–577.

Souma, J. A., D. C. Niejadlik, S. Cottrell, and S. Rankel. 1973. Comparison of thyroid function in each trimester of pregnancy with the use of triiodothyronine uptake, thyroxine iodine, free thyroxine, and free thyroxine index. Am. J. Obstet. Gynecol. 116:905–910.

Sturgeon, P. 1956. Iron metabolism. Pediatrics 18:267–298.

Svanberg, B., B. Arvidsson, A. Norrby, G. Rybo, and L. Solvell. 1975. Absorption of supplemental iron during pregnancy—a longitudinal study with repeated bone-marrow studies and absorption measurements. Acta Obstet. Gynecol. Scand., Suppl. 48:87–108.

Thompson, R. H. S., and D. Watson. 1949. Serum copper levels in pregnancy and in pre-eclampsia. J. Clin. Pathol. 2:193–196.

Tovey, L. A. D., and G. H. Lathe. 1968. Caeruloplasmin and green plasma in women taking oral contraceptives, in pregnant women, and in patients with rheumatoid arthritis. Lancet ii:596–600.

Underwood, E. J. 1971. Trace Elements in Human and Animal Nutrition, 3rd ed. Academic Press, Inc., New York. 543 pp.

Valberg, L. S., J. Sorbie, W. E. N. Corbett, and J. Ludwig. 1972. Cobalt test for the detection of iron deficiency anemia. Ann. Intern. Med. 77:181–187.

von Studnitz, W., and D. Berezin. 1958. Studies on serum copper during pregnancy, during the menstrual cycle, and after the administration of oestrogens. Acta Endocrinol. 27:245–252.

Vought, R. L., and W. T. London. 1965. Estimation of iodine excretion in nonhospitalized subjects. J. Clin. Endocrinol. Metab. 25:157–163.

Wayne, E. J., D. A. Koutras, and W. D. Alexander. 1964. Clinical Aspects of Iodine Metabolism. Blackwell Scientific Publications, Oxford.

Wolf, W. R., W. Mertz, and R. Masironi. 1974. Determination of chromium in refined and unrefined sugars by oxygen plasma ashing flameless atomic absorption. J. Agric. Food Chem. 22:1037–1042.

Zak, B., H. H. Willard, G. B. Myers, and A. J. Boyle. 1952. Chloric acid method for determination of protein-bound iodine. Anal. Chem. 24:1345–1348.

Contributors

ROY W. BONSNES, Department of Obstetrics and Gynecology, The New York Hospital-Cornell Medical Center, New York, New York

K. MICHAEL HAMBIDGE, Department of Pediatrics, University of Colorado Medical Center, Denver, Colorado

ROBERT H. KNOPP, Department of Medicine, Harborview Medical Center, and Associate Director, Northwest Lipid Research Clinic, Seattle, Washington

ALVIN M. MAUER, Medical Director, St. Jude Children's Research Hospital, Memphis, Tennessee

AGUSTIN MONTES, Catedra 2, de Fisiologie, c/o J. Tamaret, Facultad de Medicina, Ciudad Universitaria, Madrid 3, Spain

ROY M. PITKIN, Department of Obstetrics and Gynecology, University Hospitals, The University of Iowa, Iowa City, Iowa

W. ANN REYNOLDS, Department of Anatomy, University of Illinois Medical Center, Chicago, Illinois

HOWERDE E. SAUBERLICH, Chief, Department of Nutrition, Letterman Army Institute of Research, Presidio of San Francisco, California

WILLIAM N. SPELLACY, Department of Obstetrics and Gynecology, University of Florida College of Medicine, Gainesville, Florida

MARIA R. WARTH, Boston, Massachusetts

195